T0327898

DRINK UP
&
GLOW

DEDICATION

For my healing witches, Dr. Kantor and Sarah Schwab, thank you for setting me on the right path. And, as always, for Iggy!

Quarto.com

© 2024 Quarto Publishing Group USA Inc.
Text © 2024 Gabriella Mlynarczyk
Photography © 2024 Nicola Parisi
Illustration © 2024 Mabel Sorrentino

Published by Fair Winds Press, an imprint of The Quarto Group,
100 Cummings Center, Suite 265-D, Beverly, MA 01915, USA.
T (978) 282-9590 F (978) 283-2742

Fair Winds Press titles are also available at discount for retail, wholesale, promotional, and bulk purchase. For details, contact the Special Sales Manager by email at specialsales@quarto.com or by mail at The Quarto Group, Attn: Special Sales Manager, 100 Cummings Center, Suite 265-D, Beverly, MA 01915, USA.

28 27 26 25 24   2 3 4 5

ISBN: 978-0-7603-8758-0

Digital edition published in 2024
eISBN: 978-0-7603-8759-7

Library of Congress Cataloging-in-Publication Data available.

Design: Amy Sly, The Sly Studio

Page Layout: Emily Austin, The Sly Studio
Cover Illustration: Mabel Sorrentino
Photography: Nicola Parisi
Photo Styling and Propping: Gabriella Mlynarczyk
Illustration: Mabel Sorrentino

Printed in China

The information in this book is for educational purposes only. It is not intended to replace the advice of a physician or medical practitioner. Please see your health-care provider before beginning any new health program.

DRINK UP
& GLOW

NON-ALCOHOLIC, ADAPTOGEN-INFUSED DRINKS FOR OPTIMAL WELLNESS, ENERGY, AND STRESS RELIEF

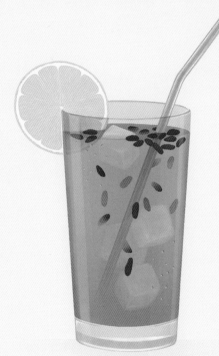

Gaby
Mlynarczyk

FAIR WINDS

Contents

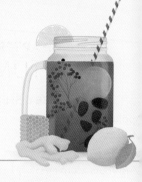

CHAPTER 1
SPRING

CHAPTER 2
SUMMER

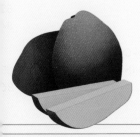

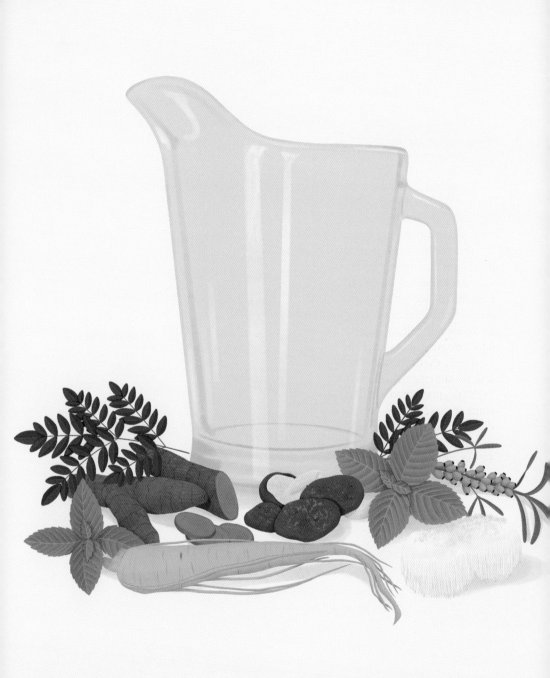

Introduction

"You are what you eat," as the saying goes. Another you might consider is "you reap what you sow." But this isn't a book of sayings or fables. More so it's a guide to help you replenish your body, sharpen your mind, and find your "glow" with nutritious, restorative, plant-based supplements, collectively known as adaptogens.

Adaptogens are herbs, roots, and mushrooms that contain phytochemicals (meaning natural chemicals occurring in plants) that have been used for centuries in alternative medicines and indigenous healing traditions, including Ayurveda and Traditional Chinese Medicine. These ancient healing modalities have been used with great success to metabolize stress, increase energy, improve brain functioning, and provide immune support. In other words, adaptogens have been healing humanity well before Western medicine was ever invented.

In fact, most Western medicines are made using many of these adaptogens re-created in synthetic form, their properties artificially amplified to suit the quick-fix culture that we humans have become incredibly reliant upon. In our modern Corporate America–driven culture, this "I'm late, I'm late, for a very important date" mentality paired with an almost manic desire to succeed and outdo our neighbors, results in anxiety, lack of sleep, depression, and sickness.

To counter this, we take fast-acting, man-made drugs, as well as other more addictive substances, to numb the pain and get us through our day-to-day lives. Obviously, the downside to a lot of these medications is that they cause some pretty intense side effects. And because Western medicine is still fairly new in comparison to the OG plant medicines, we're still discovering what the long-term effects of some of these may be. Consider the reasons some well-known, over-the-counter digestive aids have been taken off pharmacy shelves. Or how about that famous painkiller that has been the subject of a class action lawsuit? The truth is, many FDA-approved medicines, more than 14,000 in fact, have been recalled in the last ten years alone.

For me, the choice is clear. To heal my body and mind, I'll stick with the plants.

MY STORY: FROM AN ENGLISH COUNTRY GARDEN TO A LOS ANGELES BAR

I grew up a first-generation Brit in a tight-knit Polish community in the middle of England. When we kids had any sort of illness, my grandmother would turn to her small back garden and whip up a tonic to help with our maladies, the way her parents and grandparents had done before her. These tisanes (a fancy term for steeped leaves in hot water) would almost immediately alleviate headaches, upset tummies, and cold symptoms. I had—still do have, actually—an intense desire to eat all the chocolate and dairy I could lay my hands on. I didn't discover until years later that I am in fact highly allergic to both. So obviously I drank a lot of Granny's concoctions, which, to mini-me, were miracle cures that fueled my lifelong fascination with all things plant medicine.

In my professional life, I spent many years working in the highly stressful world of hospitality, as both a line cook in kitchens that depend on the high intensity production of well-plated food, and as a bartender, server, and later manager, juggling multiple orders, dealing with irate humans, and performing fast-paced, ever-changing problem-solving on the go.

Unsurprisingly, the long hours and late nights—not to mention the culture of the New York and L.A. bar scenes from the 2000s on—resulted in me becoming susceptible to overuse of alcohol and painkillers to get me through a shift. (My Polish granny and her healing plant tonics seemed a long way away at this time.) At one point as a nightclub manager, I inhaled a whole bottle of tequila in a forty-eight-hour time frame. That's twenty-six shots that I'm not particularly proud of consuming, but at the time I couldn't see my way out of that rat race lifestyle of late to bed, early to rise, rinse and repeat.

One such binge caused me to lose my eyesight in one eye at the tail end of a busy Friday night. I was convinced I'd had some sort of stroke and sought medical help of the Western kind. By the time my appointment came around my sight had returned, but the well-meaning, and quite confused doctors decided they wanted to give me an endovascular aortic biopsy (yes, it's as scary as it sounds), as well as a spinal tap to determine the root cause of this frightening episode.

Not having the funds to afford American health care, I seriously considered moving back to the U.K. to get diagnosed. As I deliberated, a good friend of mine whose opinion I highly respected, recommended that I visit her holistic healer who specialized in chiropractic kinesiology (the science of movement). He had helped heal her and her young daughter. He also used naturopathic, herbal medicines to help rebalance out-of-whack musculature and brain functioning.

It had been a while since I'd tried anything plant-based, but I had nothing to lose at this point, so I placed myself in his patient hands. He immediately told me to quit drinking alcohol, eating sugar, and smoking cigarettes, as well as recommending a change in job to lessen the stress on my body, brain, and heart. I immediately went cold turkey on everything but my job and began to see positive results within a couple of weeks.

To help with everyday stressors, I took a formula called Rescue Remedy, a combination of herbs, flowers, and roots including pine, honeysuckle, and gentian to help calm my thoughts. Once he was assured I responded well to this, I moved on to milky oat extract for higher octane stresses. Gotu kola, turmeric, ginseng, and licorice were introduced to assist with immune function, depleted adrenals (caused by stress and long days), inflammation, and energy levels. When I was feeling under the weather, licorice root and elderberry along with maca were my superhero, cold-fighting sidekicks.

With his prescriptive recommendations, I had more energy, slept better, reduced my anxiety, improved my immunity, and lost weight as the cherry on the sugar-free cake. Suffice to say, I started to feel like I was glowing again.

The downside of these adaptogenic remedies is that they can taste quite intense, so I started tinkering with dropping them into my daily beverages. I took cues from that most famous British nanny (the one with the bottomless carpet bag) and added a (metaphorical) spoonful of sugar to help the medicine go down. Pretty soon, I was mixing up adaptogenic smoothies and shots, tonics and tinctures, punches and pitchers, lattes and lemonades, and many, many mocktails (or NO-cktails, as I prefer to call them). I took my years of experience mixing up craft cocktails and designing high-end drink menus based on local, seasonal ingredients and unique, chef-inspired flavor combinations, lost the alcohol, artificial sugar, and most of the caffeine, and added my new botanical best friends. Now I make drinks that make people feel great for more than just a night. And I want to help you do the same.

Twenty years on from that first health crisis, I have continued to use adaptogens daily and now rarely seek a Western medical practitioner's help. In my opinion, adaptogens are the secret to that healthy glow everyone's looking for and can almost never permanently find. It's my hope that the recipes in this book will help you better understand these amazing plants and how they can aid in metabolizing stress, reducing anxiety, and restoring cognitive brain function, and how they can give you the good, steady energy you need to thrive every day.

HOW TO USE THIS BOOK

My aim with this book is to give you a solid blueprint of how to incorporate adaptogens into your daily life, presenting them in recognizable formats such as smoothies or nonalcoholic cocktails inspired by old-school classics such as margaritas and juleps.

Before we get into the recipes, I've provided a list of all the adaptogens featured in this book, from A to Z. While not a complete list of every adaptogen out there, it does include my best recommendations and all the ingredients I use for my restorative beverage recipes. Each ingredient includes a synopsis of its benefits as well as symbols to give you an at-a-glance view of how they can help you.

I've also included a list of tools and equipment I, as a professional bartender, could not live without, because many of my recipes involve some simple cooking. Fear not, there's nothing much more complicated than boiling water, blending a smoothie, or juicing an apple.

The book is laid out in four seasonal recipe chapters, each of which features the flavors and produce that are appropriate and available for that time of year. Each chapter is further broken down into drinks based on the time of day.

- Drinks filed under **Rise & Shine**, for example, are best for morning consumption: smoothies, lattes, etc.

- **Lunchtime Aperitifs** I chose for midday because noon is about the time when your digestive enzymes begin to dwindle, causing heartburn and bloating. The beverages in this section all contain powerful digestion aids, such as ginger and lemon, as well as adaptogenic ingredients that will assist in stomach enzyme production.

- As for **Afternoon Glow Shots**, these are shots that include just enough adaptogenic oomph to get you through the rest of the workday. Each includes a brain booster and energy booster to tackle that afternoon slump, and serotonin and immunity boosters for that feel-good factor.

- **Chill Pills & Nightcaps** are more appropriate for evening enjoyment, and include a few mocktails as well as soothing and relaxing beverages to help you wind down and get ready for bed.

- Finally, each chapter includes a couple recipes for **Drinks for a Crowd**: nonalcoholic pitchers and punches for parties and other special occasions.

Each season features twenty recipes that utilize adaptogens and pairs them with both pantry and farmers' market staples, some of which you might have to hunt for depending on where in the world you live, but most should be available at your local market or online. I hope that these recipes inspire you and help you find a path to rebalance your life and find your glow.

To your health!

An A-to-Z Guide to Everyday Adaptogens

Below is a list of every adaptogen used in this book, a description of what they do, and any applicable safety warnings. The symbols are designed to help you understand at a glance the benefit of each adaptogen.

➕ **DIGESTIVE HEALTH & IMMUNE SUPPORT**

🧠 **BRAIN FUNCTION & FOCUS**

🔋 **ENERGY & ENDURANCE**

🧑 **ANXIETY & STRESS RELIEF**

A NOTE ON MEASUREMENTS & DOSAGES

You will notice throughout the book that most of the adaptogens are measured out in very small quantities such as 0.7 milliliters (about 0.02 fl oz or 14 drops). Annoyingly, most measuring jiggers start at 5 milliliters (about 0.17 fl oz). To measure these minute quantities, rely on the pipette from the bottle (most of the adaptogens are listed in their liquid form) or use a measured eyedropper. You can find one easily online; they usually start at 0.25 milliliters (about 0.008 fl oz), and go up to 1 milliliter (about 0.03 fl oz).

In general, you should be following the dosage amounts listed on the packaging. These can vary depending on the manufacturer, so please always check the packaging and do not exceed the recommended dosage.

DISCLAIMER

The adaptogens listed in this book are safe for human consumption; however, consult with your doctor before starting any new supplemental regimen, especially if you are pregnant or nursing, have been prescribed any medications, have any sort of diagnosed disease or allergies, etc.

ALBIZIA

Albizia is used primarily for anxiety and stress, thanks to its sedative qualities. It also helps tame a sore throat and upset stomach (runny tummy). This is found most commonly in liquid form.

SAFETY CONSIDERATIONS: Do not use when pregnant.

AMLA

This gooseberry-like fruit is native to India and China, and it is widely used in Ayurvedic medicine. It is believed to be a sort of fountain of youth, helping with longevity and cognitive brain function. It is also rich in vitamin C.

ASHITABA

Great for brain function and aiding in focus, this plant calls Japan its native home, where it is revered as an ingredient full of antiaging properties, as well as for digestion and immunity. It is a good source of vitamins B_6 and B_{12}.

ASHWAGANDHA

This MVP of adaptogens is used often in Ayurvedic medicine to support the immune system and promote sleep, as well as being a superhero combatant of everyday stress. This plant regulates the stress hormone cortisol and helps when you're feeling run down or overwhelmed. It is also a powerful antioxidant.

SAFETY CONSIDERATIONS: Do not take this supplement if you are pregnant or allergic to nightshades.

ASTRAGALUS

Less of a tension tamer and more of a whole-body support system, astragalus protects from disease and inflammation, as well as assisting with digestion and recovery from illness. This adaptogen is one of the most used ingredients in Traditional Chinese Medicine.

SAFETY CONSIDERATIONS: Do not use when pregnant or breastfeeding.

BACOPA

Bacopa is traditionally used in Ayurvedic medicine to help with brain function, focus, and learning, and is often prescribed for patients with attention deficit hyperactivity disorder (ADHD) and Alzheimer's disease. It helps restore dopamine and serotonin levels and can also combat anxiety.

SAFETY CONSIDERATIONS: Do not use when pregnant or breastfeeding, or if you have heart disease.

BAOBAB

This fruit from the baobab tree is highly nutritious and is an excellent electrolyte, helping replenish lost minerals on hot sunny days and during exercise. It also aids in increasing energy levels. Like any fruit, it should be eaten in moderation, as too much can give you tummy upset. Baobab is a good source of vitamin C, zinc, magnesium, and calcium.

BURDOCK ROOT

Used in Traditional Chinese Medicine for centuries, burdock root contains tannins and sterols. It is used to lower high glucose levels in the blood, fight infections such as the common cold, and detox the blood.

Burdock root is also an antioxidant that helps mitigate the effects of free radicals, fighting inflammation and assisting with autoimmune disorders. It is also a powerful diuretic.

BUTTERFLY BLUE PEA FLOWER

This ingredient is popular with mixologists for its beautiful deep blue color that changes to amethyst when mixed with acid, but it is also a great ingredient for enhancing focus and relieving stress. Used in both Chinese and Ayurvedic medicine for centuries, it has all manner of extra health and beauty benefits including collagen production and helping with hair loss.

CHAGA

Considered a parasite to birch trees, this mushroom originates in Eastern and Northern Europe. It has been used for centuries as an immune booster, for overall health, and to help tame stress as well as increase energy levels. It is also considered a powerful anticarcinogen that helps fight certain cancers.

SAFETY CONSIDERATIONS: May interfere with blood clotting. Do not take if allergic to mushrooms.

CORDYCEPS

These days cordyceps is now farmed using soybeans as the host (sparing the lives of many a ghost moth) as it has become one of the most sought after adaptogens for its benefits of increasing muscle energy, endurance, and immune support.

SAFETY CONSIDERATIONS: Do not take if allergic to mushrooms.

ELDERBERRY

In comparison to some of the other adaptogens presented here, elderberry, or sambucus as it's often called, is only good for immune support. But I included it because it is such a powerhouse, able to knock out the flu and assist in lowering blood pressure. It is chock-full of vitamins C, A, B_6, and minerals such as iron and potassium. Rich in antioxidants, the humble elderberry can prevent wrinkles and reduce inflammation.

A WORD OF WARNING: Raw elderberry contains high concentrations of cyanide, so make sure to cook them fully before consuming.

SAFETY CONSIDERATIONS: Do not consume raw or if you are pregnant or breastfeeding.

GINSENG (AMERICAN)

American ginseng, not to be confused with other forms of ginseng, is probably the most accepted adaptogen in modern society, known to stimulate libido in men and tame menopause symptoms in women. It is also a powerful stimulant and increases energy rapidly. Great for endurance as well as increasing focus, the downside of this is that it can also elevate heart rate and cause tummy upset. I recommend taking this in dropper form.

This is one adaptogen where it is best to start with low doses and work up slowly to higher amounts.

SAFETY CONSIDERATIONS: Do not take without consulting a physician if you are taking any heart medications. Do not take if pregnant or breastfeeding.

GINSENG (SIBERIAN)

Technically not from the same family as other ginsengs, Siberian ginseng is called so for its beneficial similarities to them. It has milder properties, does not cause palpitations, and can give you a good boost of energy to get through long worknights. Because of this, it's a supplement that can be used for longer periods of time without resulting in "the jitters."

Siberian ginseng is also a useful supplement for heart health and reducing cholesterol as well as for immune support.

SAFETY CONSIDERATIONS: Do not take without consulting a physician if you are taking any heart medications.

GOJI BERRY

Goji berries are high in essential amino acids; in fact, they contain all nine of them! High in vitamin C, it's a great adaptogen to take for immune support and as an anti-inflammatory as well as being a great supplement to increase energy levels. One of my favorite ways to take goji berries is to soak them in filtered water and blend them into a refreshing pink spicy limeade that I take when I'm on the go. (Yes, recipe is in here!)

SAFETY CONSIDERATIONS: Do not take if you are allergic to the nightshade family.

GOTU KOLA

Used for thousands of years in Chinese and Ayurvedic medicine to heal wounds, treat skin conditions, and improve mental clarity, gotu kola is the little herb that could. Gotu kola is high in a compound that makes it very useful to heal wounds, used often to treat psoriasis or burns, and prevent scarring. These same chemicals reduce anxiety and increase mental function as well as treat insomnia.

As with many adaptogens, start slow with gotu kola and gradually increase the dose, but do not take every day. I personally will take this adaptogen for one month on and one month off. Speak with your holistic doctor or practitioner or health care provider to determine the best dosage for you.

HOLY BASIL (TULSI)

Long used as a treatment for bronchitis, this adaptogenic herb is also great as an immune booster, antiviral, and mood enhancer. Unlike other adaptogens that require an accumulation of doses to bring about their full benefits, holy basil acts instantly, relieving stress and alleviating depression as well as taming seasonal allergies. My favorite way to use it is as part of a salad or in a delicious tea.

LION'S MANE

Used in Traditional Chinese Medicine for centuries to treat royalty, the lion's mane mushroom boasts a plethora of benefits including boosting concentration, increasing mental clarity, taming depression, and helping to heal wounds, as well as offering immune support. Most often taken in capsule form, lion's mane is also available in a dropper bottle and as a coffee.

SAFETY CONSIDERATIONS: Do not take if allergic to mushrooms.

MACA

I first encountered maca about ten years ago when I was suffering from a terrible cold that would not shift. A trendy juice bar offered me a maca boost in my smoothie and it almost immediately alleviated my symptoms due to its high potency of vitamin C. Now, when I have a cold, it's my first line of defense. Not only is it great for immune support, but it also works as a mood enhancer, boosts libido, and is a powerhouse of essential minerals such as magnesium, calcium, potassium, and iron.

MORINGA

Moringa leaf contains high levels of tryptophan, the amino acid that sends you to sleep after eating your Thanksgiving turkey dinner. It helps boost serotonin levels in the brain for that feel-good factor and is also a great supplement to take for aiding digestion, lowering cholesterol and blood sugar, and for antiaging. Contains high levels of vitamin B_6 and vitamin C.

NETTLE

Turns out that pesky weed that used to sting your legs as you ran through it as a kiddo is an important adaptogen rich in vitamins A, B_1, B_2, C, and K, and minerals calcium, copper, and magnesium. It's useful in supporting the immune system and the adrenals when your stress levels are high. Steep the leaves in water for a soothing tea.

PINE POLLEN

Pine pollen is the only plant that contains the hormone DHEA, a compound that is a mood enhancer, libido elevator, immunity booster, and powerful anti-inflammatory. When we're run down from overwork, our DHEA gets severely depleted, so keeping pine pollen on hand for when our schedules get busy is a must. Pine pollen also serves as a good supplement to help reduce cholesterol and tame a hangover.

Because DHEA is a hormone, it's important to keep dosages of this adaptogen on the lower side and talk to your doctor before using if you have any hormonal imbalances.

REISHI

Reishi mushrooms have been used for centuries in Traditional Chinese Medicine to boost immunity, elevating white bloods cells that fight infection and taming allergies as it balances histamines. Reishi also works to calm nerves and alleviate anxiety and depression, helps with sleep disorders, increases energy levels, and lowers blood sugar levels. The common way to take reishi as a supplement is in capsule and dropper form.

SAFETY CONSIDERATIONS: Do not take if allergic to mushrooms.

RHODIOLA

I first encountered this supplement years ago when it was better known as golden root. I would take it to increase my energy on busy weekend shifts when I was on my feet for up to fourteen hours a day! Rhodiola helps with endurance; it's often used by athletes in training. It also strengthens your body's response to psychological and physical stress and helps increase serotonin levels, improving sleep, mood, and appetite.

Like most adaptogens, it's necessary to build up a certain level of the supplement before seeing benefits; usually within a week you will notice a difference. Follow daily dose recommendations on the brand that you buy and, as always, consult with your herbal health practitioner when deciding on the dosage that is right for you.

SCHISANDRA BERRY

A wonderful source of vitamin C, schisandra berries are commonly used to help with cognitive health, depression, and stress. They also help the body resist the effects of anxiety and support the body's defense against illness. The berries are said to be helpful for high blood pressure. As a menopausal woman, I also use schisandra berries to help tame symptoms such as hot flashes and heart palpitations.

SAFETY CONSIDERATIONS: Do not use when pregnant or breastfeeding. Can cause stomach irritation if taken in too large a dose.

SEA BUCKTHORN

Sea buckthorn is rumored to be the only plant containing all four omega fatty acids. Its oil includes an acid that is also found in human skin, which helps heal wounds quickly. Sea buckthorn oil is also high in vitamins, minerals, and antioxidants to support your health and immunity.

Because of its plentiful omegas, it improves cholesterol levels and reduces blood pressure as well as blood sugar.

SHATAVARI

Shatavari, a member of the asparagus family, is considered a beneficial herb to help your body cope with physical and emotional stress. It is also a potent antioxidant. I personally use shatavari to help with my wicked menopause symptoms and as an aid in fighting fatigue.

Shatavari is available in both dropper and capsule form.

SHIITAKE

As well as being a delicious, flavorful mushroom used in cooking, shiitake mushrooms are also used in Traditional Chinese Medicine to promote virility, energy, and youthfulness. Shiitake mushroom extract is also fantastic for immune support, helping with the cold and flu, recovery from certain cancers, lowering cholesterol and blood sugar levels. It is also rumored to be a powerful aphrodisiac.

Dried shiitake mushrooms are my preference for cooking and teas, but for immune support, I usually take the capsule form.

SAFETY CONSIDERATIONS: Do not take if allergic to mushrooms. Do not take when pregnant or breastfeeding.

TURMERIC

One of my personal favorite adaptogens! This root has high levels of curcumins and is a powerful antioxidant and anti-inflammatory. Curcumins are beneficial for brain function, improving moods and helping to release serotonin into the blood stream. I most often take turmeric in powdered form, but I will also juice it for my favorite wintertime treat, the Golden Latte. You can also steep the root for turmeric tea that can be enjoyed iced or hot.

VELVET BEAN (*MUCUNA PRURIENS*)

Velvet bean has been used in Ayurvedic medicine for centuries to help promote sleep. Velvet beans contain L-dopa, the precursor molecule to dopamine, which elevates levels of pleasure and enhances moods.

It is also said that velvet beans help with the treatment of Parkinson's disease, though it is not recommended to eat it in high quantities. Because the bean is a psychoactive (it has the same properties as coffee except for the addiction factor), it also helps with focus, mental clarity, and energy.

Kitchen Essentials for Making Great Drinks

While I've deliberately designed the recipes in this book to be approachable for all readers, a few basic kitchen tools are necessary to make deliciousness happen! Fortunately, whipping up adaptogenic drinks doesn't require anything too fancy or super expensive. (A Nutribullet works just as well as a pricey Vitamix blender.) I realize it's not always possible to afford a veggie juicer, however many towns have fresh veggie juice stores where you can pick up a cup of carrot juice for a few dollars.

Because most people will already be familiar with these tools, I'm including my recommendations for the best versions of these products on the market, including both "splurge" and "steal" options, so there's something that works for everyone.

GADGETS

BLENDER

STEAL: The Nutribullet personal blender, with its small footprint and powerful motor—powerful enough to chop ice into tiny shards—is the go-to blender for many a smoothie maker. As a bonus, the top comes off and can be used as a cup on the go, meaning less clean up and more convenience. At one point I turned my nose up at it, but after experiencing its durability, I am born again! You can find the personal models for around $40 to $50.

SPLURGE: The queen of blenders and the envy of many a culinarian is the Vitamix. This baby has multiple speeds, is great for pureeing and chopping everything from ice, baby food, smoothies, soup, and homemade nut butter. The downside is the price tag; the average cost is $400.

CARBONATOR

STEAL: The Phillips Soda Streaming machine is another gadget with a small footprint. It can fit onto most countertops without being in the way and also fits most budgets too at around $55 or so. You can use it to carbonate water, teas, juices, and cocktails, but beware: when CO_2 and citrus meet, you're likely to see an eruption akin to Mount Vesuvius. Avoid this by not filling the carbonator bottle past the halfway mark.

SPLURGE: More mid-price than a splurge, the Drinkmate OmniFizz carbonating system is probably my favorite tool for carbonating beverages. It's powerful and

PRO TIP

To get super crisp bubbly liquid, store it in the fridge for a few hours before zapping with CO_2. The gas adheres better to cold liquids than room temp.

creates just the right amount of crisp in your bubbles. The price tag is around $200, which might seem like a lot, but when you compare it to some of the pricier models out there (I'm talking $700), the Drinkmate is a bargain and works far more efficiently.

CITRUS JUICER

STEAL: I have a Cuisinart Pulp Control Citrus Juicer that has gotten me through countless special events and produced juice quickly. For $28 or so, this is one of the MVPs of my home kitchen, and as a bonus, it doesn't take up too much storage space.

SPLURGE: The Breville Citrus Press Pro electric juicer is my pick here, mostly for its ability to crank out juice efficiently and offer an easy clean up. There are more expensive citrus juicers out there, such as the Omega C-20C, which would set you back about $400, but its more time consuming to take apart and clean up. Not worth it in my opinion.

MILK FROTHER

STEAL: I have two suggestions here. First is the Magic Wand from the Modernist Pantry. Sleek and stylish, it whips up liquid (and cappuccino foam) effortlessly. My second choice is the Café Casa Milk Frother, which I am never without when behind the bar. Both are priced under $20. Use them for mixing up syrups and adding powdered adaptogens to your beverages; they make short work of getting everything incorporated nicely

SPLURGE: If you're serious about silky latte foam, then the Subliminal NanoFoamer Handheld Milk Frother is a must-have. This professional barista tool can be yours for just under $60 or so.

STICK (IMMERSION) BLENDER

STEAL: The Mueller Ultra-Stick Hand Blender makes quick work of blended soups and smoothies. This baby has nine speeds—most stick blenders have two, if you're lucky. It also comes with a bonus milk frother. At around $30, it's definitely worth having in your tool drawer.

SPLURGE: The All-Clad Cordless Hand Blender charges in a dock so you don't have that pesky cord getting in the way. If it played a tune while it blended, I would buy this $230 blender in a flash!

SLOW VEGGIE JUICER

When it comes to juicers, I strongly recommend picking a slow, cold press, masticating juicer. The spinning juicers might extract more but generate a lot of heat, resulting in juice you essentially must gulp down within fifteen minutes of making it. A slow juicer offers much less nutrient loss, meaning you can make more juice and store it in the fridge for up to three days.

STEAL: Amzchef masticating juicer is the one I've had most success with. Its relatively small compared to other slow juicers, and while clean up takes a little longer, it produces delicious, flavorful juice. You can find it on Amazon for just under $100.

SPLURGE: The Omega slow masticating juicer is the beast of cold press juicers and looks sleek and modern on your countertop. It's great for juicing large batches, but the downside is the hefty price tag.

TOOLS

TEAPOT OR CAFETIÈRE

My favorite way of steeping herbs in hot water is in a large teapot with a built-in strainer or in a cafetière French press coffee maker (you know, the pitcher with the plunger). As much as my British roots dictate I should use a classic teapot, I've lately been using an insulated, stainless-steel French press to make my daily tea brew, as it traps all those pesky little leaves and ensures that they stay in the pot. Plus no need for that old-school tea cozy your granny favored. You can find them as low as $15 online.

JIGGER

Another essential tool of my trade is a graduated jigger. It has five sets of measurements in one jigger ranging from ½ ounce (14 ml) to 2½ ounces (74 ml), I use them when mixing cocktails and NO-cktails and for measuring liquid extracts. My favorite ones are from Barfly and OXO.

MEASURING CUPS

For larger portions I use a measuring cup with both cups and milliliters; these are indispensable when creating large batches of syrups and infusions. My preference at home is a Pyrex glass measuring cup.

MESH STRAINERS

I have two picks here, the smaller one is the bartender's friend called a coco strainer, I love the ones from Cocktail Kingdom. For larger straining tasks, I use the Cuisinart strainer; as a bonus, they often have bundles of small, medium, and large strainers for under $15.

COCKTAIL STRAINER

After shaking your NO-cktails or mocktails, you will need to strain them when pouring them into your glass. This is especially important for beverages with mint leaves, cucumber slices, etc. My MVP here is the Koriko Hawthorne strainer from Cocktail Kingdom. Its tightly wound coil prevents anything from escaping into your glass.

MIXING SPOONS

Any sort of long-handled spoon will do for our purposes in this book, an iced tea or sundae spoon works just as well as a fancy bar spoon. But if you want to pick up a cocktail mixing spoon, my recommendation is the one from Hiware that you can find online. For something with a bit more weight, try any of the options from Cocktail Kingdom.

SHAKING TINS OR MASON JARS

As a professional bartender, I've always shaken beverages in the classic two-part shaking tins from Koriko, because they have a nice heavy bottom, make a good seal, and keep my cocktails cold. However, when I am home, I often use a screw-top mason jar for single drinks. Find one with a wide mouth that holds around 12 ounces (355 ml).

ICE MOLDS

If you want your iced beverages to not dilute super quickly, especially in summer, I recommend investing in some silicone ice cube trays. The larger cubes (2 × 2 inch [5 × 5 cm]) last much longer and don't water down your drinks as quickly as the smaller cubes from your freezer.

SAUCEPAN

Generally I use a good-quality, heavy-bottomed, stainless-steel saucepan with a well-fitting lid, especially when I am steeping something like cinnamon syrup, but whatever you have on hand will do.

ZEST PEELER

OXO Good Grips has a nice sturdy Y-shaped peeler that works well for creating lemon and orange twists. Choose the professional peeler because you'll get a nice thick peel, essential for spritzing over your beverages. You can also use one of those stainless-steel cheese slicers for a thicker peel.

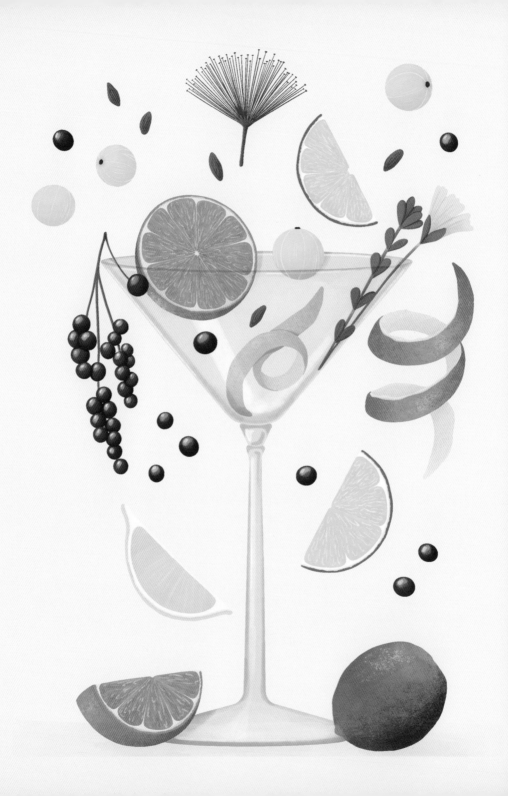

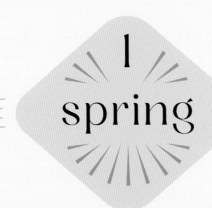

spring

Spring is the perfect time for a reset. We clean our houses, start craving lighter fare in our diets, and begin feeling the urge for movement and being outdoors. With all this activity, the brain and its functionality can sometimes get a bit neglected. We plod along in our routines, neglecting the one part of our body that can make us feel really better.

Adaptogens can help you see the world in a different, brighter light, giving you that "glow" of health and vitality you're looking for. Many of them actively help raise serotonin levels, blowing away winter blues and brain fog, making us see and think more clearly. They can also help with energy levels. After a few months of cozying up by the fire and dealing with colder weather, you might need a little help acting on your instincts to get out and move your body. Coffee and energy drinks can only do so much—and they come with side effects. Adaptogens are the better way to go, gradually increasing your serotonin and energy levels over time, and helping reset your brain.

With some adaptogens, the effects are cumulative, so it might take a few weeks before you feel the gray clouds parting in your head. Others, such as turmeric and holy basil, act almost immediately, giving you an instant burst of cerebral sunshine to lift your spirits.

Spring is also the time of year when farmers' markets refresh and become more alive, burgeoning with fresh greens, herbs, and produce. In the recipes that follow, I picked a few of my favorite springtime flavors and paired them with a selection of superhero restorative adaptogens to help you on your journey of spring awakening.

Matcha, Matcha, Matcha!

Matcha is a Japanese shade-grown green tea that is dried and ground into a powder. The fact that it's shade-grown is one of the things that makes matcha special; most other green teas, which usually come from China, are grown in full sunlight. Use culinary grade matcha or the more expensive ceremonial grade—either will work for this recipe.

In my riff on a matcha latte, I use makrut lime leaf syrup to bring a floral note to the cup. Makrut lime leaves are used in Thai and Indian cooking to infuse coconut milk in curries, and they can be found in most Asian markets or online. The adaptogen superhero here is pine pollen, known for its brain-boosting, immune-supporting, and energy-inducing properties. On a side note, it's also a powerful aphrodisiac—do with that what you will!

FOR THE MAKRUT LIME LEAF SYRUP

10 medium to large makrut lime leaves

1 cup (8 oz or 235 ml) freshly made hot simple syrup (see Note, page 34)

FOR THE MATCHA, MATCHA, MATCHA

1 teaspoon matcha green tea powder

1 cup (8 oz or 235 ml) oat milk or milk of your choice

½ teaspoon unrefined coconut oil

1 ounce (30 ml) Makrut Lime Leaf Syrup

½ teaspoon pine pollen powder

FOR SERVING

Lemon or orange peel, for oil spritzing

--- **YIELD: 1 LATTE** ---

TO MAKE THE MAKRUT LIME LEAF SYRUP: Steep the leaves in simple syrup in the fridge for up to 48 hours; the longer you leave them infusing, the fuller the flavor. Store in an airtight container in the fridge for up to 2 weeks.

TO MAKE THE MATCHA, MATCHA, MATCHA: Add all the ingredients to a small heavy-bottomed saucepan and set it on the stove over a low heat. You don't want to burn the milk, so low and slow is the best way to heat this through. I usually find about 3 minutes does the trick.

As the milk warms up, use your milk frother to gradually incorporate the matcha and pine pollen powders into the milk. Be careful to not allow the whisk to hover on the surface of the liquid, as this will cause splashes.

Once the milk is heated through and the powders are whisked in, start frothing the milk by lowering and lifting the frother into the liquid. This adds air and makes the latte frothy.

TO SERVE: When your latte is fully frothed, pour it into a cup of your choice. Spritz a lemon or orange peel over the top for some added aroma.

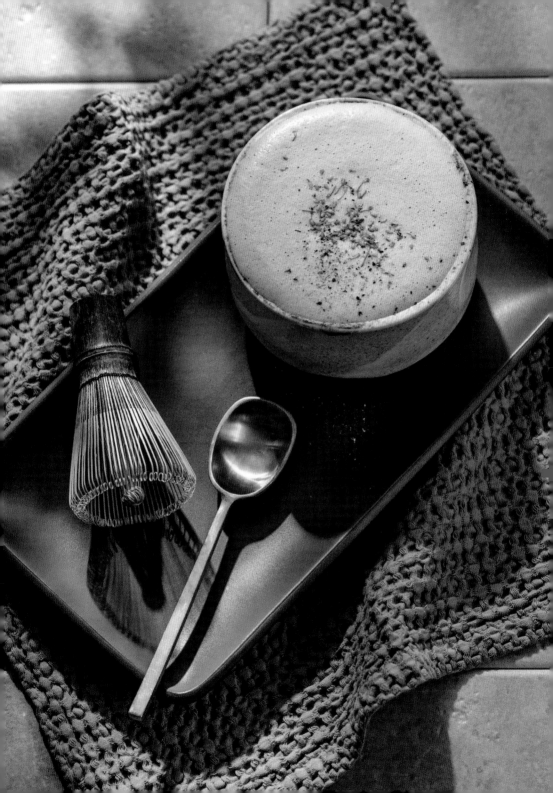

Jolly Green Rhodiola Smoothie

This smoothie is one of my all-time favorite ways to get my nutrients on the go. It's great for giving you a jolt of energy for your morning run, hike, or walk and, as a bonus, won't fill you up too much. The baobab adds prebiotics to your digestive system, setting you up for a later breakfast, while the rhodiola brings you mental clarity, kicks anxiety and depression to the curb, and boosts your energy levels. As for chlorella, this all-natural algae or seaweed is packed full of essential vitamins and minerals, and it will assist in boosting energy levels, as well as support fat loss. Can't get enough leafy greens into your diet? Try a hit of chlorella.

As for non-adaptogens, avocado adds healthy fats and a lovely gelato-like smoothness to the mix, while banana and coconut provide potassium and electrolytes to help you with your morning workout. Occasionally I'll add some shredded coconut to the mix too, for extra bulk and flavor.

Also, I should note . . . as a Brit, I'm not super fond of cold beverages, so I don't include any ice in my smoothies. Cold drinks in general are not great for your digestive tract, but if you wish to make this smoothie colder, I recommend freezing your peeled bananas instead of adding ice. Just remember, any ice will dilute the flavors here, so you might have to add more sweetener if you choose to go this route.

1 ripe avocado

1 ripe banana

½ ounce (15 ml) unrefined coconut oil

1 tablespoon (3 g) powdered chlorella

½ ounce (15 ml) honey, Grade-A Vermont maple syrup, or date syrup

1 tablespoon (7 g) baobab powder

1 milliliter (20 drops) rhodiola extract

4 ounces (120 ml) virgin coconut water

Pinch of sea salt

YIELD: 1 SMOOTHIE

Add all the ingredients to your blender and pulse until everything is smooth and incorporated. Depending on the size of your banana and avocado, you may need to add more liquid to make this smoothie slurpable.

NOTE
You can also add some peanut butter or cocoa powder to this, as well as collagen powder. In the summer, I add mixed berries or peaches for some variety.

Shiitake Almond Mocha Roca

This caffeine-laced latte is essentially a souped-up riff on the traditional café mocha with some extra flair added to it.

Shiitake is our superhero adaptogen here, known in Traditional Chinese Medicine to promote virility as well as energy and to be a powerful immune booster. Paired with flavonoid-rich cacao, which improves blood flow to the brain and the heart, this dynamic duo is sure to become your "best part of waking up."

This mocha is inspired by the flavors of Almond Roca candy, but instead of the classic toffee, I've chosen to sweeten this tasty morning beverage with maple syrup, and finish it with a pinch of Chinese five-spice powder in place of the usual cinnamon you find on coffee drinks.

1 cup (8 oz or 235 ml) almond milk or milk of your choice

1 ounce (30 ml) espresso

1 teaspoon cacao powder

1 ounce (30 ml) Grade-A Vermont maple syrup (optional)

Pinch of sea salt

2 milliliters (40 drops) shiitake extract

Pinch of Chinese five-spice powder, for serving

YIELD: 1 MOCHA

Add all the ingredients to a small heavy-bottomed saucepan and set it on the stove over a low heat. Slowly heat up the milk and as it warms up, use your milk frother to start incorporating the cacao powder into the milk. Be careful to not allow the whisk to hover on the surface of the liquid, as this will cause splashes.

Once the milk is heated through, about 3 minutes, and the powder is whisked in, start frothing the milk by lowering and lifting the stick blender into the liquid to make it frothy.

TO SERVE: Pour into a cup of your choice and sprinkle with a pinch of Chinese five-spice powder.

NOTE
This can also be made into an iced latte; just make sure the cacao is well blended before cooling and pouring over ice.

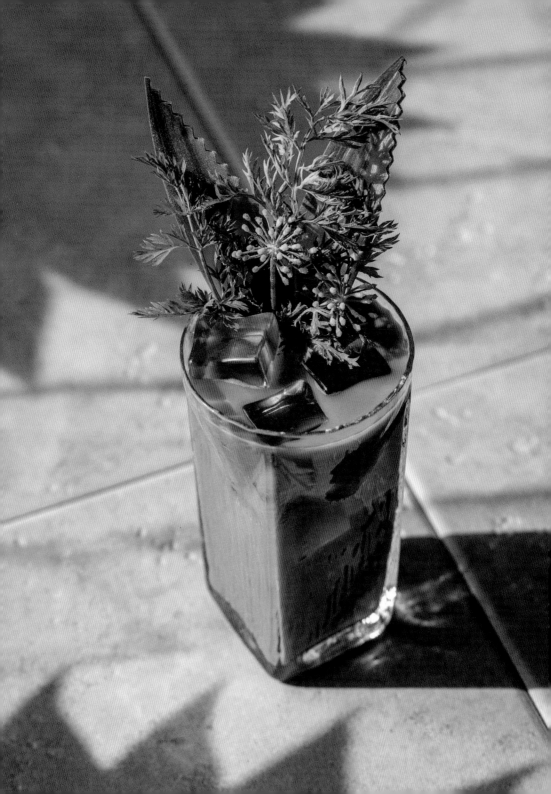

Carrot Coconut Shake with Siberian Ginseng

Back in 2011, I got to work with a very well-known Top Chef. This guy was a genius—he taught me how to pair ingredients and bring complexity to my cocktails. One of the most unexpected flavor pairings that I tried while working with him was carrot and coconut plus yuzu juice for some acidity. Yuzu is a super fragrant Japanese citrus that is a cross between a mandarin and a lemon. If you can't find yuzu, substitute lemon or orange juice instead.

This unusual culinary pairing is the backbone to this "milkshake." It shares the glass with Siberian ginseng, known to promote alertness as well as muscle-building and endurance. To add a wee kick, I included ginger juice; I usually juice it with my carrots. Vanilla rounds the whole thing out, making this one crushable shake.

3 ounces (90 ml) fresh-pressed carrot juice

2 ounces (60 ml) full-fat coconut milk

1 scoop coconut milk–based ice cream (optional)

½ ounce (15 ml) yuzu or lemon juice or 1 ounce (30 ml) fresh-squeezed orange juice

½ ounce (15 ml) ginger juice

1 milliliter (20 drops) Siberian ginseng extract

1 ounce (30 ml) date syrup or honey

1 drop real vanilla extract

YIELD: 1 SHAKE

If you have a blender or milkshake maker, add all the ingredients and pulse until frothy.

Alternatively, use a mixing bowl and a stick blender: Add the ingredients to the bowl, and place a stick blender in all the way to the bottom. Pulse a few times, holding onto the bowl so that it doesn't spill.

Pour into your glass of your choice and enjoy!

PRO TIP

If using a stick blender, place your bowl on a damp cloth to prevent it from moving around on your kitchen counter.

NOTE

I like to squeeze an orange peel over my shake before blending, expressing the orange oils out of the peel and adding the beautiful invigorating aroma of this sunshine citrus. I also add a pinch of freshly grated nutmeg when I feel particularly festive.

Goji Berry Rhubarb Sour

At this point in the book, I'm going to let you in on a secret: Spring is actually my favorite time of year. It's the time of new life, longer, sunnier days, and bright colors on display at the market. One of the most vibrant colors on display this time of year comes from the deep pink rhubarb stalks that wink at me as I wander by. When I see this beautiful bounty, I can't resist picking a few pounds up to make delicious rhubarb lemonade.

Along with our featured energy-boosting adaptogen, goji berry, the rhubarb and lemon in this recipe provide a multitude of benefits. Rhubarb contains antioxidants that are great for skin health, vitamin K for bone health, and lots of fiber and compounds called sennosides that help with digestion. The fresh-squeezed lemon juice brings that bright, refreshing tartness to the mix while balancing your tummy as its acid turns to an alkaline after you drink it.

If you can't find goji berry juice, buy dried goji berries, soak them in water, and then blend the whole shebang up in your blender. (This is actually much less expensive than store-bought juice.) Bonus, this recipe can be used to create an adaptogenic, booze-free riff on a classic Ramos fizz—see the Pro Tip!

FOR THE RHUBARB CONSOMMÉ

2 cups (280 g) chopped rhubarb (see Notes, page 34)

2 cups (16 oz or 475 ml) water

1 cup (200 g) cane sugar

½ of a vanilla bean pod (optional)

continued on next page

YIELD: 1 SOUR

TO MAKE THE RHUBARB CONSOMMÉ: Add all the ingredients to a large, heatproof bowl and stir to make sure the sugar completely coats the rhubarb. Wrap the bowl completely several times with plastic wrap (the underside too), so that any steam gets trapped inside the bowl instead of escaping. Place the bowl on top of a heavy-bottomed pan half-filled with water. The bottom of the bowl should completely cover the opening of the pan but not be sitting in the water.

continued on next page

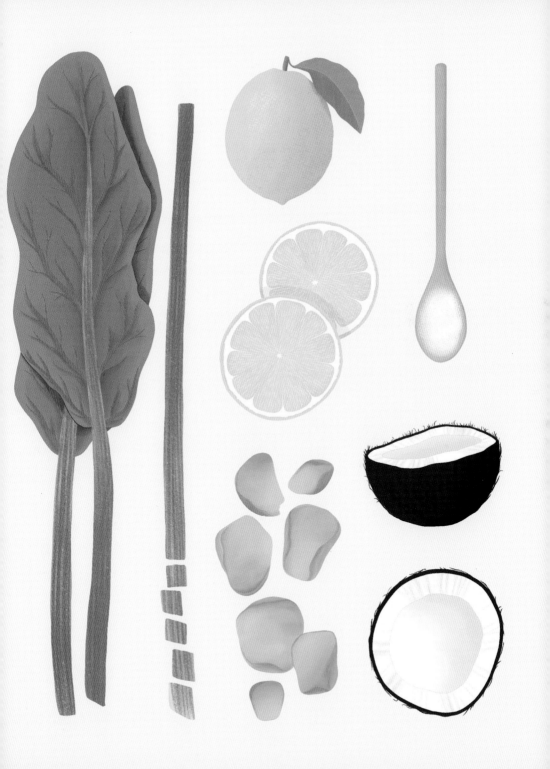

FOR THE GOJI BERRY RHUBARB SOUR

2 tablespoons (30 ml) Goji Berry Juice (page 55)

2 ounces (60 ml) Rhubarb Consommé

1 ounce (30 ml) fresh-squeezed lemon juice

2 to 3 ounces (60 to 90 ml) virgin coconut water or filtered water

¾ ounce (22 ml) simple syrup (see Notes)

1 drop rose water, such as Al Wadi brand (optional)

FOR SERVING

Lemon twist, for garnish (optional)

Bring to a simmer over medium heat, then turn the heat down to the lowest flame or setting and allow the rhubarb to steam for about 2 hours. Remove the pan from the heat and allow it to cool before straining the juicy water out of the bowl.

TO MAKE THE GOJI BERRY RHUBARB SOUR: Add all the ingredients with 3 to 4 ice cubes to your cocktail shaker or mason jar with a lid. Shake hard for 5 seconds.

TO SERVE: Pour into a chilled highball glass and fill with more ice if needed. Garnish with a lemon twist, if desired.

PRO TIP
Use this recipe as a base for a booze-free Ramos fizz. Just substitute 1 ounce (30 ml) of coconut milk and 1 ounce (30 ml) of aquafaba for 2 ounces (60 ml) of coconut water. Shake as usual, and top with sparkling water once the mix is added to the glass.

NOTES
Stored in an airtight container in the fridge, the rhubarb consommé should last up to 2 weeks.

When buying rhubarb, look for the pinkest stalks possible for the sweetest flavor and brightest color; green rhubarb stalks tend to be tarter than pink ones.

When making the consommé, I like to keep the rhubarb pulp to use in pies and cakes (but that's another book entirely).

To make the simple syrup: Mix equal parts cane sugar and hot water, stirring until the sugar dissolves completely. Allow to cool before using.

Shatavari "Salty Dog"

As a Brit, I'm partial to a bitter ale, which is why I gravitate toward hoppy IPAs as my beer of choice. But because I don't drink booze anymore, I'm always on the lookout for tasty alternatives that can satisfy my cravings. Not so long ago, nonalcoholic beer was considered a bit of a joke, but luckily some of the best breweries in the world are now producing top notch no-ABV beers, including some well-known brands such as Heineken and Brooklyn Brewery.

One particularly popular British beer cocktail is the shandy, a fizzy combination of beer and some kind of soft drink or juice. My personal favorite shandy is made by combining a hoppy IPA with grapefruit. If I can find oro blanco grapefruits, or their similar-tasting siblings, pomelos, I'll juice those, but I find the more accessible ruby grapefruit does the trick too.

This recipe also features gentian tincture, a common ingredient in Italian aperitifs, to add a touch of bitterness. This hoppy, bitter version of a Salty Dog highball is just the trick to help me wake up my taste buds and get those digestive juices flowing, while shatavari gives me the energy and serotonin boost I need to get through the rest of my workday.

0.7 milliliter (14 drops) shatavari extract

1 to 2 drops gentian tincture

2 to 3 ounces (60 to 90 ml) fresh-squeezed grapefruit juice

½ ounce (15 ml) honey or Grade-A Vermont maple syrup (see Notes)

1 drop real vanilla extract or Fiori di Sicilia (see Notes)

Pinch of sea salt, plus more for the rim (optional)

3 ounces (90 ml) nonalcoholic IPA or pilsner

YIELD: 1 APERITIF

Add all the ingredients, except the nonalcoholic beer, to a chilled glass and stir to combine with a long-handled spoon. This will make sure the salt dissolves evenly before you add the beer.

Add ice to the glass and top with nonalcoholic beer of your choice. Give a couple more stirs with the spoon and enjoy.

NOTES

To make the honey or maple syrup, mix equal parts hot water and honey or syrup. Stir until the sweetener dissolves into the water. I like to make a big batch of this and stash it in the fridge for when I need it.

Fiori di Sicilia is a delicious blend of vanilla and bright citrus that avid bakers—like myself—often sub for vanilla in their recipes. You can often find it on the same shelf as your favorite extracts or online.

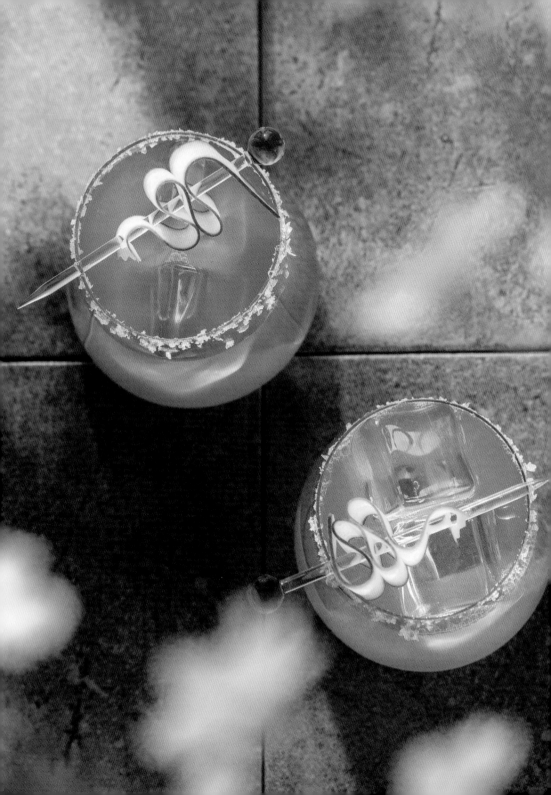

Ashitaba Jalapeño "Margarita"

A margarita without tequila (or, for my preference, mezcal) is technically an agua fresca, a refreshing beverage found on street carts in Mexico and Central America that consists of water, juice, lime, and sugar. This book includes several recipes in this vein, but since I like to add some margarita-esque touches to my adaptogenic riffs on these drinks, I feel justified in referring to them as "margaritas."

For this veggie-forward version, I start with jalapeño-infused water. Jalapeño peppers are an edible powerhouse of nutrition, chock-full of capsaicin, which is beneficial in maintaining healthy blood flow, as well as helping to regulate blood sugar levels.

As for adaptogens, the ashitaba in this recipe provides a dose of B_6 and B_{12} that will help with focus and energy levels, as well aid digestion.

The recipe is for a pitcher-size batch, which makes four to five servings and will keep in the refrigerator for a few days. The dosage of ashitaba should come out to about 1 gram per serving—so make sure you adjust this if you tinker with the serving size.

FOR THE ASHITABA JALAPEÑO "MARGARITA"

4 to 5 grams ashitaba powder (depending on serving)

3 cups (405 g) chopped cucumber

1 cup (100 g) chopped celery

3½ cups (28 oz or 840 ml) jalapeño-infused filtered water (see Notes)

4 ounces (120 ml) honey syrup (see Notes)

4 ounces (120 ml) fresh-squeezed lime juice

2 ounces (60 ml) dirty olive brine (optional)

Pinch of sea salt per serving

FOR SERVING

Tajín and sea salt, for the rim (optional)

Cucumber or lime wheel, for garnish

YIELD: 1 PITCHER OR 4 TO 5 DRINKS

TO MAKE THE "MARGARITA": Add all the ingredients to your blender and blend on high for 10 to 15 seconds.

TO SERVE: Strain through a fine-mesh strainer if you don't want pulpy bits, or pour directly into a Tajín-and-salt rimmed, ice-filled glass. Garnish with a cucumber or lime.

NOTES

To make jalapeño-infused water, use 1 chopped jalapeño per 3 to 4 cups (24 to 32 oz, or 705 to 940 ml) water. Add the jalapeño to the water, cover and infuse in the fridge for 6 to 24 hours.

"Mind Embracer" Lion's Mane Mule

This tasty, caffeinated riff on a classic Moscow mule will be just the jumpstart you need to get through a sluggish afternoon. Mules come from a category of OG cocktails called Bucks, named so because the spice from the ginger delivers a kick like a bucking mule.

In this recipe, lion's mane, known for its mental clarity, brain-boosting, and anxiety-relieving properties, pairs up with spicy ginger beer to help with digestion and with espresso or cold brew for an after-lunch energy hit.

1 milliliter (20 drops) lion's mane extract

1 ounce (30 ml) espressoor cold brew

4 ounces (120 ml) ginger beer

½ ounce (15 ml) Grade-A Vermont maple syrup (optional)

Pinch of sea salt, to cut the bitterness of the coffee

Lemon twist, for serving (optional)

YIELD: 1 DRINK

Add all the ingredients to a chilled highball glass and stir a few times to incorporate. Add ice cubes and garnish with a lemon twist if desired.

Gotu Kola Cola

Gotu kola, the magical adaptogen hero in this recipe, is abundant with superpowers, among them helping with cognitive health, stress, anxiety, and depression. In Traditional Chinese Medicine, it is considered to be the herb of longevity, promoting liver and kidney health as well as healing skin.

The glow shot below is straightforward. I pair the gotu kola with Mexican Coca-Cola because it contains real sugar as opposed to the high fructose corn syrup found in American-made cola. The classic sidekick to cola is lime juice or a lime wedge, which helps cut some of the sweetness of this soft beverage.

2 milliliters (40 drops) gotu kola extract

2 ounces (60 ml) Mexican Coca Cola

Pinch of sea salt (optional)

1 lime wedge

YIELD: 1 SHOT

In a small glass, add the gotu kola, cola, and sea salt (if using). Squeeze the juice from the lime wedge into the glass and drink!

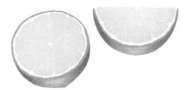

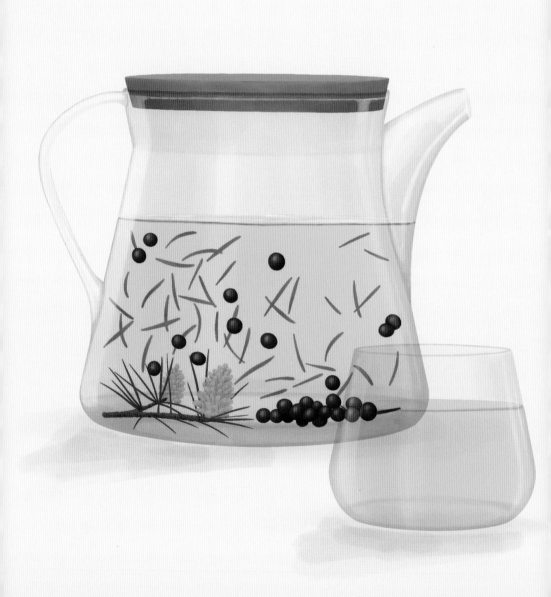

Silver Needle Schisandra Shot

As the day goes on, I always think it's better for the body to get its energy boosts from softer forms of stimulants. That is why I chose silver needle tea, a beautifully fragrant white leaf tea from China, as well as schisandra berry and pine pollen for this recipe. Both adaptogens work extremely well to promote endurance, as opposed to jolts of high energy.

I usually steep the tea in batches and store it for a few days so I can sip when needed. Pine pollen and schisandra berry also help with immunity, and the antioxidants in the tea help to promote wellness and heart health.

2 ounces (60 ml) hot or cold silver needle or other white tea

½ ounce (15 ml) honey syrup (see Note)

2 milliliters (40 drops) schisandra berry extract

2 milliliters (40 drops) pine pollen extract

Orange peel, for oil spritzing

YIELD: 1 SHOT

In a small cup, add the tea, honey syrup, and extracts. Stir until the honey syrup is well incorporated.

Spritz the orange peel over the tea and sip for a soothing afternoon pick-me-up.

NOTE
To make the honey syrup, mix equal parts runny honey and hot water until the honey is dissolved. Store in an airtight container in the fridge.

Maca Garden Greens Shot

This recipe features a widely misunderstood garden herb that often gets used as garnish and discarded to the side of the plate. I'm talking parsley, of course! When we're battling a cold, the most common advice is to OD on vitamin C. Good advice, but what if I told you that oranges contain only a fraction of the vitamin C contained in common old parsley, which is chock-full of calcium too?

Joining parsley in this immune-boosting shot is nettle for its abundance of vitamins and minerals, as well as the adaptogen maca for its mood-enhancing superpowers.

Unless you have a cold press juicer, I recommend drinking this shot as soon as you've juiced it to retain the highest level of nutrients possible. They tend to dissipate the longer this shot is left out.

½ cup (48 g) flat-leaf parsley with stems chopped off

½ cup (48 g) fresh stinging nettles (see Note)

1 medium Fuji or other sweet apple, chopped in half

¼ ounce (8 ml) apple cider vinegar

1 milliliter (20 drops) maca extract

1 drop real vanilla extract

YIELD: 1 SHOT

Add the parsley and nettle into your juicer first then feed in the apple and apple cider vinegar. The liquid from the apple will wash the remnants of the herbs through the juicer blades, ensuring you receive the maximum amount of nutrients. Stir in the maca and vanilla and drink immediately.

NOTE
They're called "stinging" nettles for a reason. Use gloves when handling them.

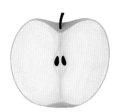

"Going for Gold!" Turmeric Shot

This shot does double duty as both a serotonin-booster and a cold-fighter from the combination of the turmeric and cayenne. As a bonus, turmeric and lemon are great digestives, assisting with the balance of beneficial flora in the gut and overproduction of acid.

I included this recipe in the Spring section because 'tis the season that I get the nastiest colds and am most in need of a drinkable cuddle.

0.7 milliliter (14 drops) turmeric tincture

1 ounce (30 ml) honey syrup (see Note)

½ ounce (15 ml) fresh-squeezed lemon juice

1 ounce (30 ml) warm water

Pinch of cayenne pepper

Lemon twist, for oil spritzing

YIELD: 1 SHOT

Add all the ingredients to a small cup and stir to allow the honey syrup to dissolve in the liquid.

Sip or shoot, but be warned—if you choose to shoot, the heat from the cayenne and the tartness of the lemon may be a little too intense at first.

NOTE
To make the honey syrup, mix equal parts runny honey and hot water until the honey is dissolved.

Ashwagandha White Grape Bianco Aperitivo

As a bartender, I always feel that one of my jobs is to find ways to help guests who abstain from alcohol not feel like they're missing out on any of the fun. The most common request I've gotten over the years is for drinks that mimic the flavor of wine. Wine is fermented grape juice, and I turn to two nonalcoholic grape-based ingredients to assist with these orders. First, verjus, which translates to "green juice," a culinary ingredient used similarly to vinegar, though without its astringency, and second, the better-known grape juice.

Using these two ingredients in tandem, along with botanical infusions, has provided me with a plethora of ideas for drinks, which I, tongue in cheek, like to call Wine-NO.

I've included a Wine-NO recipe in every chapter of this book. For my springtime recipe, which is inspired by a wine-based bianco aperitivo, I've added superhero adaptogens ashwagandha, for its calming properties that help promote sleep, and moringa, to help with anxiety and blood pressure. I've also made use of non-adaptogenic L-theanine, which helps with stress relief and stops your brain overprocessing, allowing for a calming end to the day.

0.7 milliliter (14 drops) ashwagandha tincture

0.7 milliliter (14 drops) moringa tincture

2 milliliters (40 drops) L-theanine extract

2 to 3 ounces (60 to 90 ml) chilled white verjus, depending on the desired tartness

3 ounces (90 ml) chilled unsweetened white grape juice

2 dashes nonalcoholic peach cocktail bitters

Meyer lemon twist or green grapes, for garnish

YIELD: 1 WINE-NO DRINK

Add all the ingredients, except the garnish, to a chilled wine glass. Stir to combine.

Spritz the Meyer lemon twist over the drink and pop in the glass for extra aroma. Enjoy your Wine-NO!

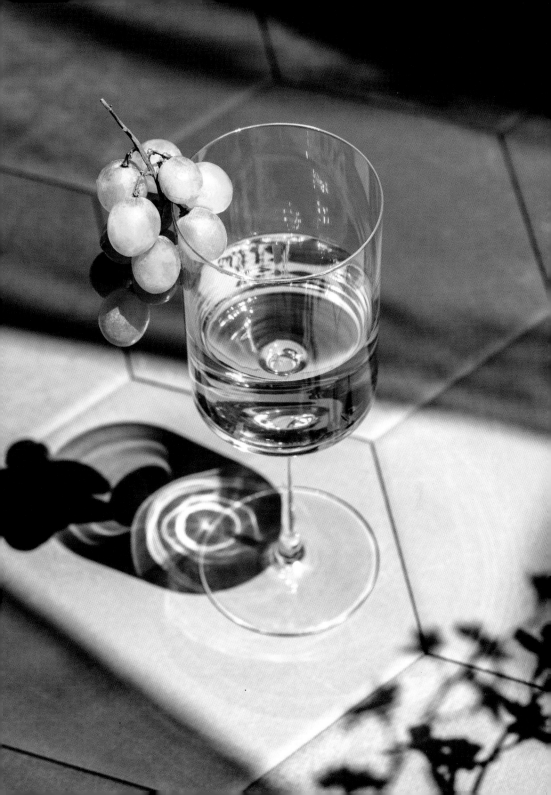

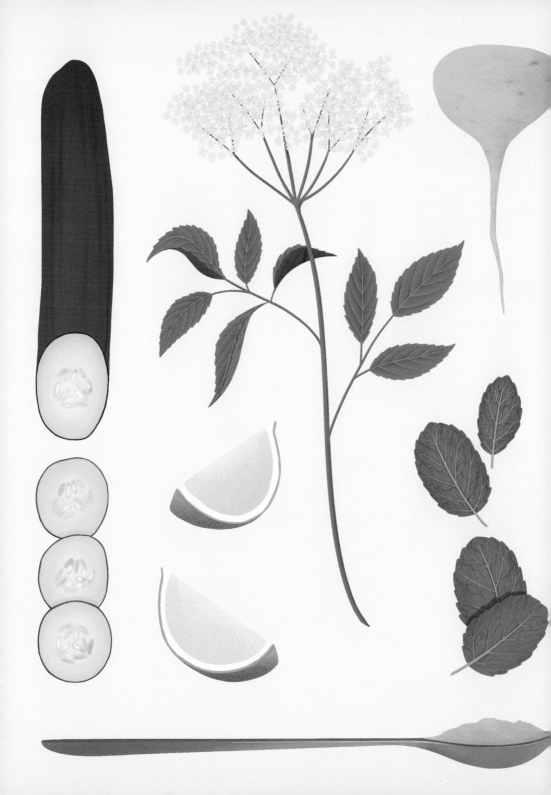

The Maca Fauxito

I have an aversion to the word *mocktail*, mostly because it conjures up the image of something overly sweet and fruity, rather than a beautifully crafted, thoughtfully balanced beverage. So, on the various menus I've created over the past fifteen years I've looked for ways (and words) to better define what it is I'm serving up.

The *fauxito*, inspired by the classic mojito, is one such example. For this particular fauxito recipe, I combine the mojito's classic key ingredient, mint, with cucumber for some refreshing complexity. In my opinion, these two are a match made in heaven. If I can find it, I like to add a nonalcoholic elderflower cordial to the mix, to make for a truly glorious spring fling. If you're lucky enough to come across fresh elderflowers, all you have to do is steep them in a solution of hot simple syrup to tease out their delicate flavors to make a sort of cordial.

My choice of adaptogen here is maca, a mood-enhancing, immune-supporting, nutrient-rich powerhouse. I promise you, you won't miss the rum at all.

5 to 6 steeped cucumber slices (see Note)

6 to 8 fresh mint leaves, plus a bushy sprig for garnish

2 to 3 lime wedges

1 teaspoon cane sugar or 1 ounce (30 ml) elderflower cordial

0.7 milliliter (14 drops) maca extract

3 ounces (90 ml) cucumber water (see Note)

2 ounces (60 ml) elderflower soda, lime sparkling water, or plain soda water

YIELD: 1 FAUXITO

Add the cucumber slices, mint, lime wedges, and sugar or elderflower cordial to a chilled highball glass. Muddle lightly by pressing the ingredients with a spoon, and stir to dissolve the sugar or incorporate the cordial into the juice expressed from the fruit during muddling.

Add the maca, cucumber water, and ice, and stir again to combine. Top with elderflower soda, lime sparkling water, or plain soda water, and garnish with a big bushy mint sprig.

NOTE
To make cucumber water, slice a cucumber and allow it to steep in filtered water for about 6 hours. Strain and use the cucumber slices for muddling in this beverage.

Burdock Bananas Foster Mai Tai

Okay, this one is a wee bit of a project and involves some cooking, so I suggest leaving it for a weekend. The classic mai tai takes its name from the Tahitian phrase meaning "the best." In this booze-free version, a creamy blend of banana, brown butter, cinnamon, and cacao makes a divine combination that, in my opinion, perfectly lives up to its name.

Burdock root and astragalus are my superhero adaptogens here, the former for its digestive support and the latter for its ability to help with immune function and recovery. Partake in this dessert-like cocktail whenever you need some yummy after-dinner comfort or just because.

FOR THE BURDOCK BANANAS FOSTER MAI TAI

1 stick (4 oz or 113 g) unsalted butter

3 extra-ripe bananas, mashed

¼ ounce (8 ml) burdock root extract

¼ ounce (8 ml) astragalus root extract

1 can (13.5 oz or 398 ml) full-fat coconut milk

3 tablespoons (16 g) cacao powder

1 tablespoon (7 g) ground Saigon cinnamon

3 to 4 ounces (90 to 120 ml) Grade-A Vermont maple syrup

¼ ounce (8 ml) orange oil

¼ teaspoon sea salt

1 to 2 scoops of ice

FOR SERVING

Bushy mint sprig

Freshly grated nutmeg

YIELD: 4 DRINKS

TO MAKE THE BROWN BUTTER: Add a stick of butter to a heavy-bottomed pan over medium heat. Allow the butter to melt, stirring it until the milk solids in the butter caramelize and turn brown. You will know when it's ready when the butter has turned an amber color. Remove the pan from the heat and stir, scraping up the brown bits at the bottom of the pan.

TO CARAMELIZE THE MASHED BANANAS: Stir them into the hot brown butter until well incorporated. The heat of the hot butter cooks the sugars in the bananas and makes them super fragrant and yummy. Allow to cool before using.

TO MAKE THE BURDOCK BANANAS FOSTER MAI TAI: Transfer your caramelized bananas, along with the butter, to your blender. Add all remaining ingredients, except the ice, and blend on high until everything is smooth and incorporated.

Add one scoop of ice and blend on high until the ice pieces become pellet-size. Taste and add more ice if needed.

TO SERVE: Transfer to chilled glassware of your choice and garnish with mint and grated nutmeg.

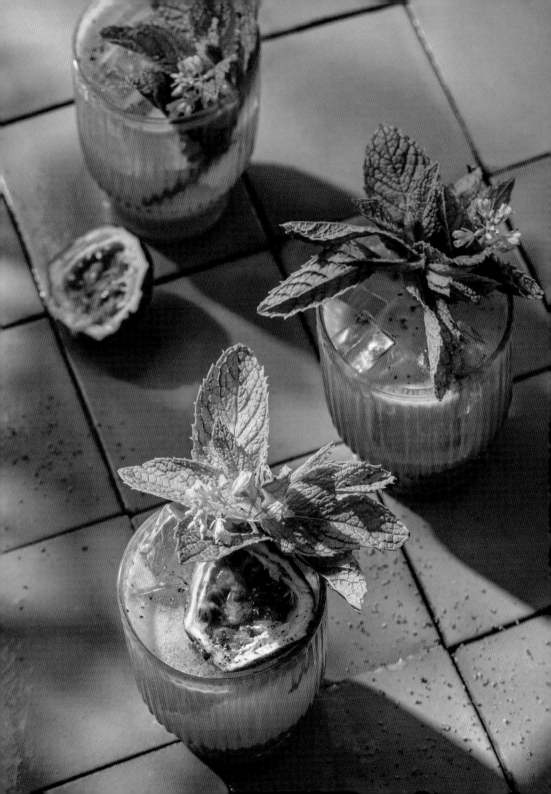

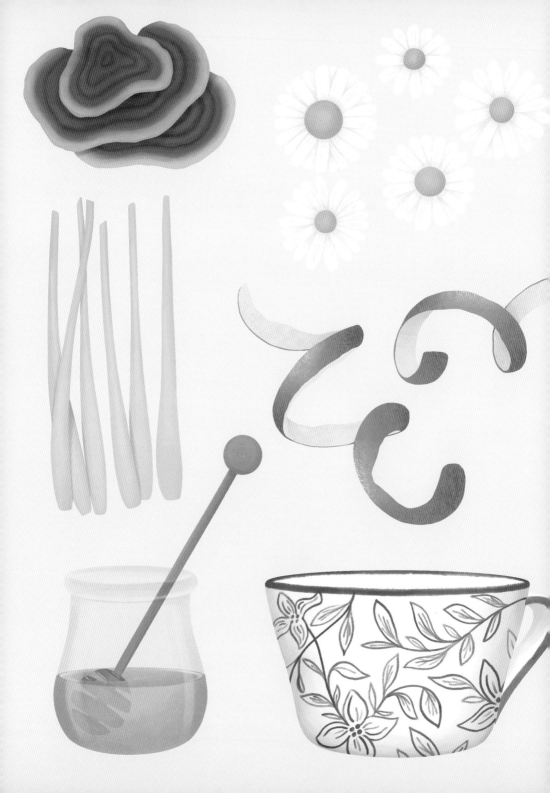

Relaxing Reishi Tisane

I first came across reishi extract several years ago during allergy season, when it was prescribed to me to help with my sniffles, runny nose, and itchy eyes. I can't say that it did a lot for my allergies, but the mental benefits it provided by targeting my anxiety and helping me sleep better made it worth it. Reishi is also a great antiviral and immune booster. In this recipe, I pair it with my favorite non-adaptogenic brain relaxer, L-theanine. Together, they have a powerful effect in this tisane, a fancy word for botanicals steeped in hot water. Enjoy it hot in a cup or chilled and over a large ice cube for a soothing nightcap.

1 milliliter (20 drops) reishi extract

2 milliliters (40 drops) L-theanine

4 ounces (120 ml) chamomile lemongrass tisane (see Notes)

1 ounce (30 ml) honey syrup (see Notes)

1 drop real vanilla extract

Orange peel

YIELD: 1 TISANE

Add all the ingredients, except the orange peel, to a cup and stir, making sure the honey is fully dissolved. Express the orange oil from the peel over the tea. Once all the oil has been expressed, plop it into the cup.

If drinking over ice, allow to cool fully before pouring into a chilled glass.

NOTES

To make the chamomile lemongrass tisane, I use a chamomile tea bag and chop up a half stick of lemongrass into the teapot and allow it to steep.

To make the honey syrup, mix equal parts runny honey and hot water until the honey dissolves completely.

Holy Basil–Cucumber Lemonade

This recipe takes full advantage of the magical powers of holy basil, an adaptogenic plant used for centuries in Ayurvedic medicine as a powerful mood tonic. Most adaptogens work overtime and cumulatively: so the more you take, the better your buzz. Holy basil works immediately to calm your anxiety and brighten your outlook, which is one of the reasons it's such a great adaptogen for parties! I've tried holy basil tea in this recipe but found that it muddies the fresh flavors of the cucumber and dill, so instead I prefer to use holy basil extract for my hit of instant sunshine in this drink.

Serve this in a tall pitcher with cucumber ice cubes for a celebratory feel.

FOR THE CUCUMBER ICE CUBES

1 cup (8 oz or 235 ml) cucumber juice

1 cup (8 oz or 235 ml) filtered water

Sliced Persian cucumbers or other smaller-size cucumbers

FOR THE HOLY BASIL–CUCUMBER LEMONADE

2.8 milliliters (56 drops) holy basil extract

3 cups (24 oz or 710 ml) cucumber juice

4 ounces (120 ml) fresh-squeezed lemon juice

4 ounces (120 ml) simple syrup (see Note)

FOR SERVING

Dill sprigs

Cucumber Ice Cubes

Lemon slices

YIELD: 4 SERVINGS

TO MAKE THE CUCUMBER ICE CUBES: Stir the cucumber juice and water together and pour it into ice cubes trays. Add 1 to 2 slices of cucumber into each mold and freeze. These will keep in the freezer for 2 to 3 weeks.

TO MAKE THE HOLY BASIL–CUCUMBER LEMONADE: Add all the ingredients to a large pitcher and stir well.

TO SERVE: Add cucumber ice cubes to each glass, along with a sprig of dill. Pour the lemonade over the ice cubes. Garnish with a lemon slice and enjoy.

NOTE

To make the simple syrup, mix equal parts cane sugar and hot water, stirring until the sugar dissolves completely. Allow to cool before using.

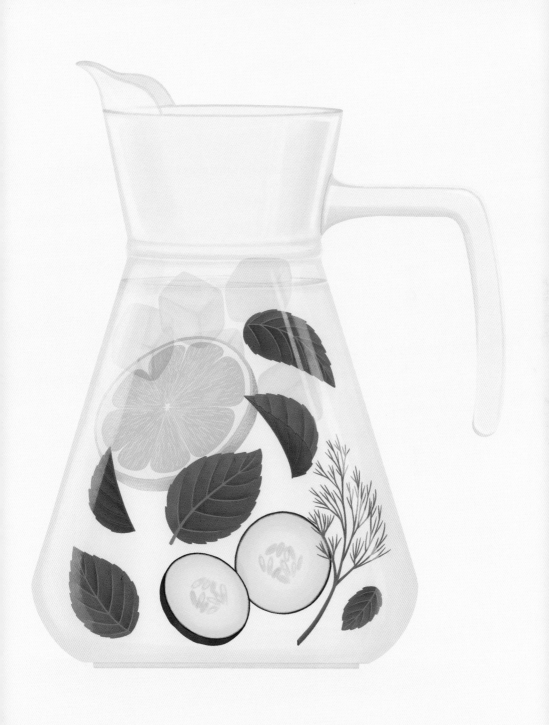

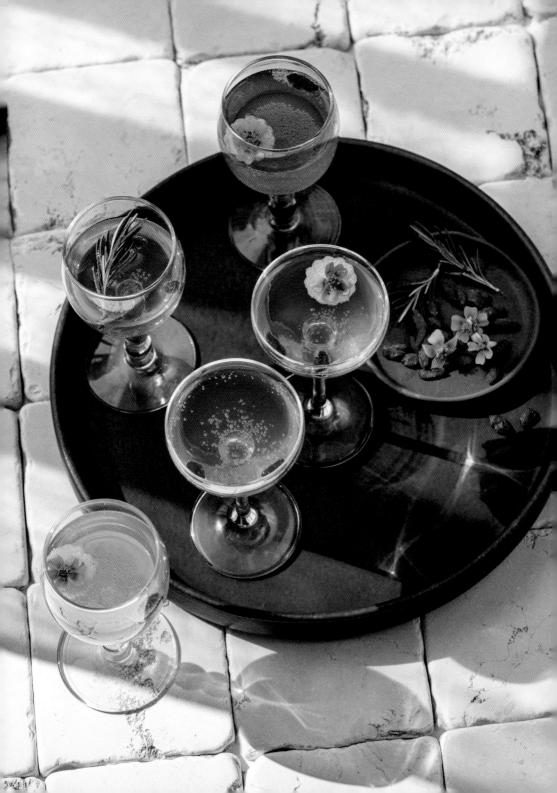

Elder Goji Berry Punch

Goji berries are well known to be high in antioxidants, and in Traditional Chinese Medicine, have been revered for thousands of years for their immune system–stimulating prowess. Often you'll see them sprinkled on top of acai bowls and sometimes on fruit salads, but it's rare that you'll find them in a beverage, because the juice is quite pricey. The dried berries themselves, however, are far more budget-friendly and are widely available in most supermarkets in the dried fruit aisle. My recipe utilizes a home-blended goji berry juice, which only requires a little planning to give the berries time to fully hydrate. I suggest soaking them overnight. Once the juice is blended up, it can be stored in the refrigerator for a few days. Just make sure to give the liquid a good stir before using.

This punch recipe also features elderberry extract and elderflower syrup for a bright, refreshing celebratory punch.

FOR THE GOJI BERRY JUICE

1 cup (106 g) goji berries

3 cups (24 oz or 710 ml) filtered water, plus more for soaking

FOR THE ELDER GOJI BERRY PUNCH

2¼ cups (18 oz or 540 ml) Goji Berry Juice or nectar

6 ounces (175 ml) elderflower syrup

1½ ounces (43 ml) alcohol-free elderberry extract

6 ounces (175 ml) fresh-squeezed lemon juice

1½ cups (12 oz or 355 ml) elderflower soda

FOR SERVING

Lemon slices

Rosemary sprigs

YIELD: 6 TO 8 SERVINGS

TO MAKE THE GOJI BERRY JUICE: Add the goji berries to a bowl and cover completely with filtered water. Let the berries soak overnight to fully hydrate. When you're ready to make the juice, strain out the water the berries have been soaking in. Add the soaked berries and 3 cups (24 oz or 710 ml) of fresh filtered water to your blender. Blend on high for about 30 seconds. Strain through a fine-mesh strainer to remove the pulp, if desired. Store in an airtight container in the fridge for up to 5 days.

TO MAKE THE ELDER GOJI BERRY PUNCH: Add all the ingredients to a punch bowl and chill. If you have limited shelf space in your fridge, you can chill it in a pitcher.

TO SERVE: Add ice and garnish with lemon slices and rosemary sprigs.

PRO TIP

If this is a special occasion, make one giant ring ice cube by filling a babka or ring mold with water and freezing it. To make it even fancier, place lemon slices, edible flowers, and dried goji berries into the water.

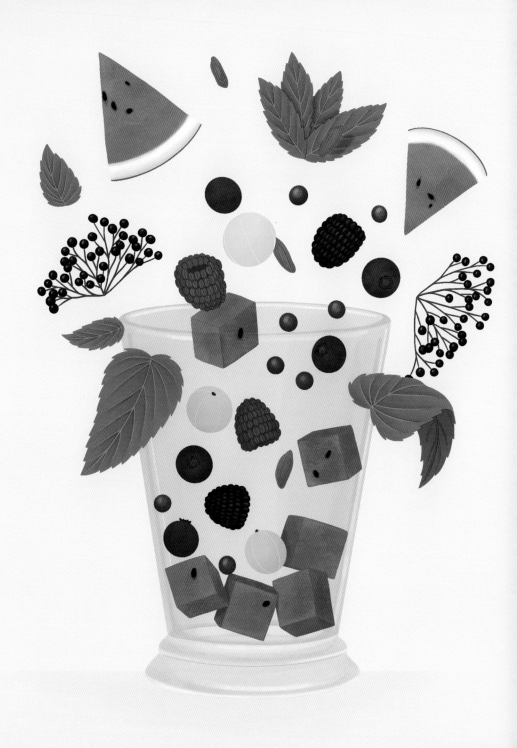

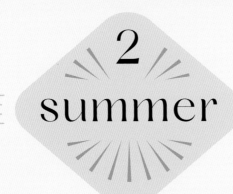

2

summer

Ah, summertime! The time of year we should be spending all day lazing in the sun and soaking up as much vitamin D as possible. Sadly, with climate change, it's often too hot (even in England!) to spend more than a couple of hours outside before running for the cover of shade.

In summer, you'll likely find yourself sweating much more, so it's vital that you hydrate with water and water-heavy fruit and veg. This is also an ideal time of year to reconsider your alcohol consumption. While a wine spritzer or pitcher of margaritas may sound like the ideal summertime drink, they will seriously deplete your hydration levels. That, in turn, will sap your brain power and energy, and can even lead to heatstroke, especially if you're hanging at the beach.

Methinks a better way of celebrating summer is to whip up some of the recipes in this chapter to keep you cool as a cucumber and sharp as a tack. What's more, summer is the time of year that all manner of delicious, flavorful produce is on full display. Just check out your local farmers' market to find soft peaches dripping with delicate nectar, watermelons full to bursting with sweet juice, and berries of all shapes and colors winking at you from their baskets.

One of my favorite ways of utilizing and prolonging this summer bounty is by making drinking vinegars or shrubs (the precursor to the modern-day soda syrups) and large batches of consommés that I keep in the freezer for use later in the year. You will find a couple of shrub recipes in this chapter and in others.

I also include in this season's offerings one of my all-time favorite summer beverages, the shandy, that thankfully these days can be made nonalcoholic with the wonderful array of NA beers that even big breweries are jumping on board with. Shrubs and icy cold beers, regardless of if they're boozy or not, are a match made in heaven and will result in something like a saison or rustic, sour beer.

And so, without further ado, I present to you summertime and some easy livin'!

Holy Rhodiola Smoothie Bowl (or Acai Bowl)

Buying a prepared acai bowl from a store will cost you a pretty penny, however, these days, you can find frozen sachets of it in most good supermarkets. It takes very little time to whip up your own, more cost-effective, smoothie or smoothie bowl.

While technically not considered an adaptogen, acai is chock-full of antioxidants and omega-3 fatty acids. It is believed to offer many benefits, including improving your heart health by lowering cholesterol and improving your cognitive function by fighting inflammation in brain cells.

In this recipe, I pair it with rhodiola, to help set you up for the day with a clear mind, and with holy basil, for that feel-good factor. Serve this up as a smoothie by adding a little more liquid, or as an acai bowl (using less liquid for a thicker consistency) topped with your favorite fruit, nuts, and seeds. If you're cow milk–challenged (like me), any plant milk or goat milk yogurt will work great in this recipe, but of course substitute with whatever type of milk you prefer.

0.7 milliliter (14 drops) rhodiola extract

1 milliliter (20 drops) holy basil extract

1 sachet (about 4 oz or 113 g) unsweetened frozen acai puree

½ avocado

1 cup (200 g) unsweetened coconut yogurt or yogurt of your choice

½ ounce (15 ml) runny honey

1 banana, sliced (for smoothie; use only ½ for a bowl)

1 cup (8 oz or 235 ml) nut milk or soymilk (optional)

½ cup (75 g) frozen blackberries

Sea salt (optional)

1 drop real vanilla extract (optional)

——— **YIELD: 1 SMOOTHIE OR ACAI BOWL** ———

TO MAKE A SMOOTHIE: Add the rhodiola, holy basil, acai, avocado, yogurt, honey, a whole banana, milk (if using), blackberries, sea salt (if using), and vanilla (if using) to your blender. Blend on high until the desired consistency is reached. Pour into a glass and enjoy!

TO MAKE AN ACAI BOWL: Add the rhodiola, holy basil, acai, yogurt, honey, half a banana, blackberries, sea salt (if using), and vanilla (if using) to your blender. Blend on high until it reaches your desired consistency. It will be thicker than a smoothie as you've omitted the milk. Scoop into a bowl, top with a selection of fruits and nuts, and enjoy!

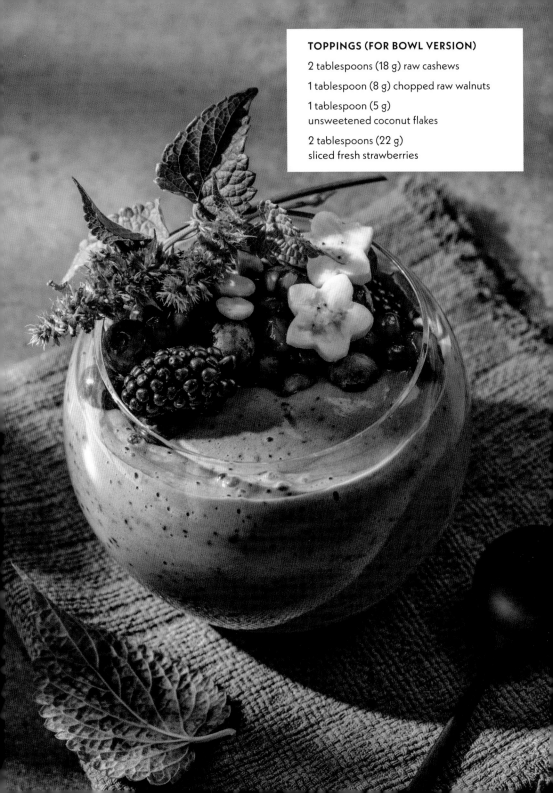

Velvet Bean Shake

If this is the first time you're trying velvet bean, get ready, because there's a good chance you won't be able to live without it after this. Sold under the name mucuna, the powder derived from these legumes can be slipped into all manner of shakes and smoothies. In Ayurvedic medicine, it has been used for centuries to manage nervous disorders, moods, cognitive function, male infertility, iron deficiencies, and more. It is also rumored to be useful for Parkinson's disease, cancer, and bacterial infections.

The velvet bean contains naturally occurring L-dopa, which is a precursor to dopamine. As well as the benefits listed above, it's also a fantastic supplement to take for energy and endurance, but be careful with your dosing. Velvet bean can sometimes negatively affect digestion, so it's best to start small and work up to using a full teaspoon.

I pair velvet bean with fresh strawberries to make an adult version of the strawberry milk I grew up loving so much. I also add a touch of rose water to the blender, bringing the beautiful aroma of an English garden into your morning drink. For a more liquid-y shake, omit the banana, which is there to provide a little bulk. As a Brit who is not fond of too much ice, I drink my shake almost at room temp, but serve yours over ice or chill it in the fridge if you prefer it cold. Or, if you like, you could add a scoop of low-sugar frozen coconut ice cream to the mix—after all, it's summer!

¼ to 1 teaspoon
velvet bean powder

½ cup (75 g) fresh strawberries

½ banana

1 cup (8 oz or 235 ml)
unsweetened oat milk
or milk of your choice

1 teaspoon rose water, such as
Al Wadi brand (optional)

Pinch of sea salt

1 drop real vanilla extract

YIELD: 1 SHAKE

Add all the ingredients to your blender and blend on high for 30 seconds. Strain through a fine-mesh strainer if you want to remove any pulp. Serve at room temperature or cold.

Schisandra Berry Peachy Palmer

This is a nontraditional way to enjoy your morning green tea buzz. In this peachy riff on an Arnold Palmer, we freeze green tea into ice cubes to use as the water substitute in this drink. Making frozen tea cubes is very straightforward. After you've steeped your tea in hot water, allow the tea to cool, then place in ice cube trays overnight so that your caffeine fix is ready for your morning commute.

You can also use other types of tea here, such as a caffeine-free rooibos or red bush tea (especially one that incorporates chai spices). White tea and black tea also work beautifully with the peach and lemon flavors in this recipe.

As far as adaptogens go, sea buckthorn and schisandra berry are working together here to provide you with a feel-good boost of anxiety relief, energy, and immune support. Bonus: They're also great for supporting glowing skin and a healthy heart.

This drink is so refreshing, I urge you not to limit it to just breakfast time. As with a regular Arnold Palmer, you can drink this one any time you like!

3 ounces (90 ml) chilled jasmine green tea or tea of your choice, plus more for ice cubes

2 milliliters (40 drops) schisandra berry extract

1 ounce (30 ml) sea buckthorn juice

3 ounces (60 ml) peach nectar (see Notes)

1½ ounces (45 ml) fresh-squeezed lemon juice

1 ounce (30 ml) simple syrup (see Note, page 34)

FOR SERVING

Lemon slices

YIELD: 1 DRINK

TO MAKE THE ICE CUBES: Steep the green tea according to package directions. When the tea is fully steeped, remove the bags and discard. Let the tea cool to room temperature. Set 3 ounces (90 ml) aside and pour the rest of the tea into an ice cube tray and place the tray in the freezer to freeze overnight.

TO MAKE THE SCHISANDRA BERRY PEACHY PALMER: Add all the ingredients, including 1 to 2 tea-laced ice cubes, to your shaker tin or mason jar with a lid. Shake hard and pour into your drinking vessel of choice.

TO SERVE: Add more tea cubes and a slice of lemon.

NOTES

Most supermarkets carry peach nectar in the juice aisle.

This recipe can be made into a pitcher for brunch, lunch, or any gathering really!

Make the simple syrup for this recipe ahead of time.

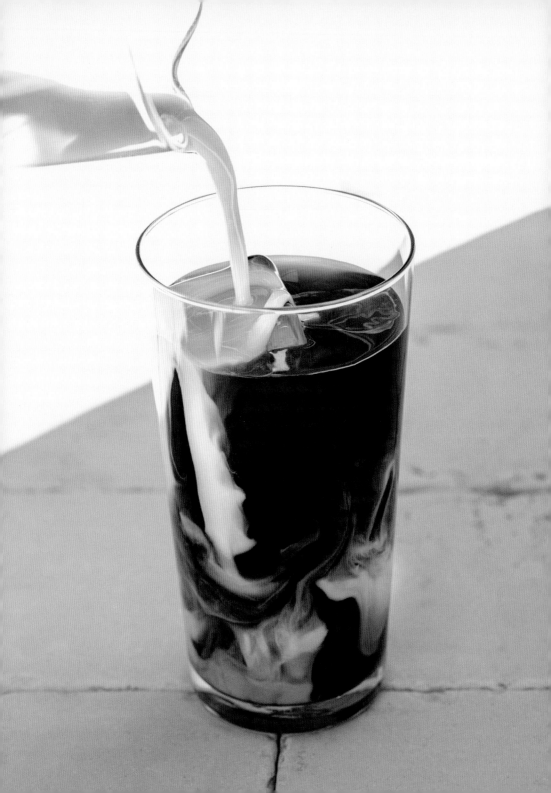

Lion's Mane Vietnamese Coffee

Vietnamese iced coffee and Thai iced tea are two of my favorite summertime guilty pleasures. Guilty in the fact that they both contain sweetened condensed milk, which brings a lot of sugar to this highly caffeinated party. However, I firmly believe that everything in moderation makes for a less dull existence.

Lion's mane, a brain-boosting anxiety fighter, is our adaptogenic superhero in this recipe. I use the liquid extract over the powder here because it blends easier—the powder in a cold drink doesn't dissolve as well. For the condensed milk, I turn it into a syrup by adding an equal amount of hot water and allowing it to cool before using. This makes it flow a little easier and cuts down on some of the sweetness. If I'm feeling festive, I'll add Saigon cinnamon sticks to the syrup to infuse while it cools.

FOR THE CONDENSED MILK SYRUP

1 cup (8 oz or 235 ml) condensed coconut milk or milk of your choice

1 cup (8 oz or 235 ml) boiling water

FOR THE LION'S MANE VIETNAMESE COFFEE

2 milliliters (40 drops) lion's mane extract

6 ounces (175 ml) dark roast Vietnamese coffee or dark roast coffee of your choice

1½ ounces (45 ml) chilled Condensed Milk Syrup

Pinch of sea salt

FOR SERVING

Cold brew or regular ice cubes

Orange twist

Ground cinnamon

--- YIELD: 1 COFFEE ---

TO MAKE THE CONDENSED MILK SYRUP: Add the milk and boiling water to a heatproof pitcher. Stir to combine. Cool before using.

TO MAKE THE LION'S MANE VIETNAMESE COFFEE: Add all the ingredients to your shaker tin or mason jar with a lid. Whip shake (see Pro Tip below) for 10 to 15 seconds to get the heavy syrup mixed into the liquid consistently.

TO SERVE: Pour the drink into your vessel of your choice and add the ice. Express the orange oil from the orange twist over your glass or cup by squeezing or twisting it. Add a pinch of ground cinnamon and go!

PRO TIP

"Whip shaking" is type of shake that uses either no ice or one small piece of ice to add air to the liquid without diluting it. This is most often used in egg white sour style cocktails. I use it in this recipe to hand froth the mix to give it a lush airy texture.

"Pinkies Out" Amla Sour

This spectacularly pink sour gets its name from both its vibrant hue and the fact that when you drink it from a coupe glass, you feel so fancy, you can't help but stick your pinky out.

    This recipe gets its adaptogenic boost courtesy of maca and amla, a dynamic duo with their mood-enhancing properties. Amla is also a wonderful digestive tonic to help with any postprandial bloat and, as the icing on the proverbial cake, also offers a boost of energy.

    I love using fresh ripe strawberries in this sweet, tart treat, which gets extra pucker-inducing love from fragrant hibiscus tea. Just make sure that your strawberries are almost on the verge of being overripe, with no green patches, or the flavor will lose some of its fullness.

YIELD: 1 SOUR

FOR THE STRAWBERRY SYRUP

2 cups (290 g) fresh ripe strawberries, leaves removed

2 cups (16 oz or 475 ml) simple syrup (see Note, page 34)

FOR THE "PINKIES OUT" AMLA SOUR

1 milliliter (20 drops) amla extract

0.5 milliliter (10 drops) maca extract

2 ounces (60 ml) chilled hibiscus tea

1½ ounces (45 ml) fresh Strawberry Syrup

1 ounce (30 ml) fresh-squeezed lemon juice

½ ounce (15 ml) simple syrup (see Note, page 34)

¼ teaspoon balsamic vinegar (optional)

Pinch of fresh black pepper

Strawberry slice, for garnish

TO MAKE THE STRAWBERRY SYRUP: Add ingredients to your blender and blitz on high for about 30 seconds. Pass the puree through a fine-mesh strainer to remove the seeds, using the back of a spoon to push as much of the syrup through as possible. (Use the seedy pulp to top off your overnight oats or acai bowl.) Store in an airtight container inthe fridge for up to 5 days.

TO MAKE THE "PINKIES OUT" AMLA SOUR: Add all the ingredients with 5 ice cubes to your cocktail shaker or mason jar with a lid. Shake hard for 5 seconds. Strain into a chilled cocktail coupe or glass of your choice and garnish with a sliced strawberry on the rim.

PRO TIP

A classic sour cocktail is usually made with some sort of frothing agent to create that beautiful cloud of foam that rests on the top of the drink. Egg white is the OG option for this, but I've long been fond of subbing aquafaba, a vegan option made from the water in a can of chickpeas. I promise it does not taste like chickpeas! For a frothier version of this drink, add 1 ounce (30 ml) of aquafaba to your cocktail shaker along with the other ingredients and shake as usual.

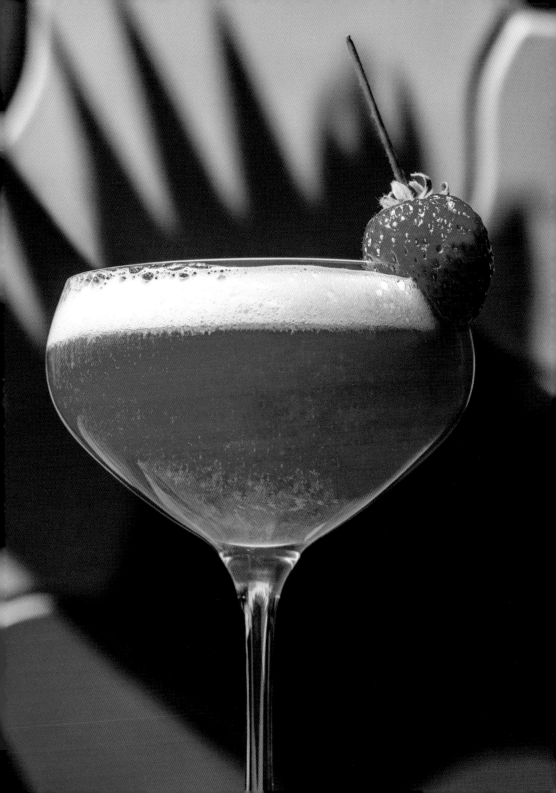

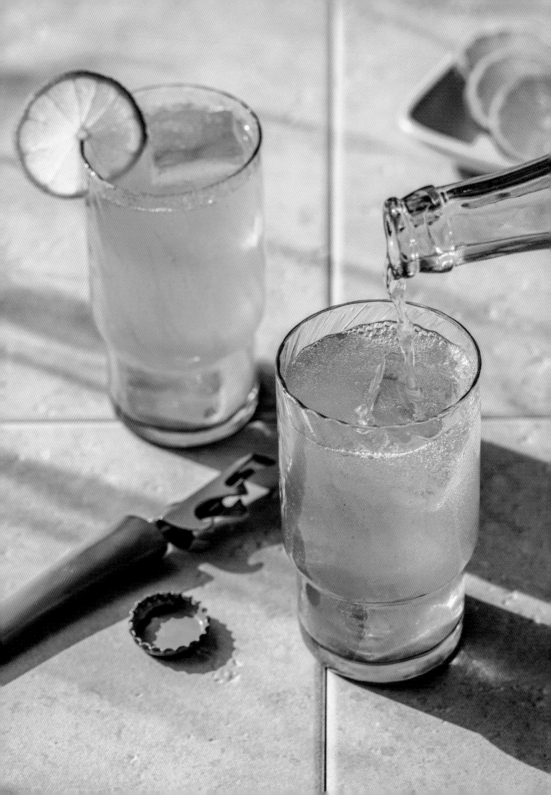

Schisandra Shandy

The classic British shandy is usually equal parts lager beer and fizzy lemon lime soda, but in Ireland they use ginger beer instead, which is my preference. The bump of apple cider vinegar brightens this mix up and provides a digestif aid.

Some of the ingredients I use in this recipe are staples of Indian cuisine, both adaptogen turmeric and fragrant curry leaves are featured prominently in many traditional dishes. Schisandra berry, with its ability to slay anxiety and boost immunity as well as endurance, and turmeric, with its mood-enhancing, antioxidant properties, are my picks for this refreshing, spicy afternoon shandy that will surely help you keep all your mind-bending dragons at bay.

FOR THE TURMERIC, GINGER, CURRY LEAF SYRUP

1 cup (240 g) peeled, chopped fresh ginger root

¼ cup (60 g) fresh peeled turmeric root

¼ cup (24 g) fresh curry leaves

4 cups (32 oz or 960 ml) simple syrup (see Notes)

FOR THE SCHISANDRA SHANDY

2 milliliters (40 drops) schisandra berry extract

1 ounce (30 ml) Turmeric, Ginger, Curry Leaf Syrup

½ ounce (15 ml) fresh-squeezed lime juice

½ ounce (15 ml) apple cider vinegar

2 ounces (60 ml) chilled dry ginger beer

4 ounces (120 ml) chilled nonalcoholic pilsner

Lime wheel or wedge, for garnish

YIELD: 1 SHANDY

TO MAKE THE TURMERIC, GINGER, CURRY LEAF SYRUP: Add all the ingredients to your blender and blitz on high for about 1 minute. Strain through a fine-mesh strainer, pushing the syrup through with the back of a wooden spoon. Store in an airtight container in the fridge for up to 2 weeks.

TO MAKE THE SCHISANDRA SHANDY: Add the schisandra berry; turmeric, ginger, and curry leaf syrup; apple cider vinegar; and lime juice to a tall, chilled glass and stir to combine. Pour in the ginger beer and stir again to remove some of the bubbles (and avoid overflow when you add the pilsner). Slowly pour chilled nonalcoholic pilsner into the glass. Garnish with a lime wheel or wedge and serve.

NOTES

If you can't find curry leaves, use a half teaspoon of good-quality curry powder, but be sure to check the ingredients label. Some of the less thoughtfully prepared ones contain garlic and onion powder, which is the last thing you want in a beverage!

Make the simple syrup for this recipe ahead of time. Mix equal parts cane sugar and hot water, stirring until the sugar dissolves completely. Allow to cool before using, and refrigerate it to store.

Holy Water "Margarita"

What better way to hydrate and stay cool in the summer than with a slice of juicy watermelon? Actually, I take that back—a slice of watermelon is the second best way. The first is this recipe for a watermelon-laced, nonalcoholic "margarita," which is so much more than your standard agua fresca.

This summer recipe is packed full of the quintessential fruit of the season and features my favorite good vibes adaptogen, holy basil, as well as ashitaba to keep your brain focused and your synapses firing full throttle through the afternoon. I've also added my secret ingredient for booze-free margaritas, olive brine, to add a touch of tequila-like vegetal flavor to this mix.

Like many of the drinks in this book, this recipe can be used throughout the day, but remember: Ashitaba can be a powerful brain stimulant. Reduce the dose or leave it out all together to feel great without the buzz!

FOR THE HOLY WATER "MARGARITA"

0.7 milliliter (14 drops) holy basil extract

1 milliliter (20 drops) ashitaba extract

3 ounces (90 ml) juice of watermelon, basil, and mint (see Notes)

1 ounce (30 ml) fresh-squeezed lime juice

¾ ounce (22 ml) chilled simple syrup (see Notes)

½ ounce (15 ml) olive brine

FOR SERVING

Tajín or sea salt, for the rim

Bushy mint sprig

Watermelon spear

YIELD: 1 "MARGARITA"

TO MAKE THE HOLY WATER "MARGARITA": Add all the ingredients with 5 ice cubes to your cocktail shaker or mason jar with a lid. Shake hard for 5 seconds.

TO SERVE: Strain into a chilled glass rimmed with Tajín or salt. Fill with ice and garnish with a bushy mint spring and watermelon spear.

NOTES

To prep the watermelon juice, add basil and mint to your juicer as you're juicing your watermelon. It's divine.

Make the simple syrup for this recipe ahead of time. Mix equal parts cane sugar and hot water, stirring until the sugar dissolves completely. Allow to cool before using, and refrigerate it to store.

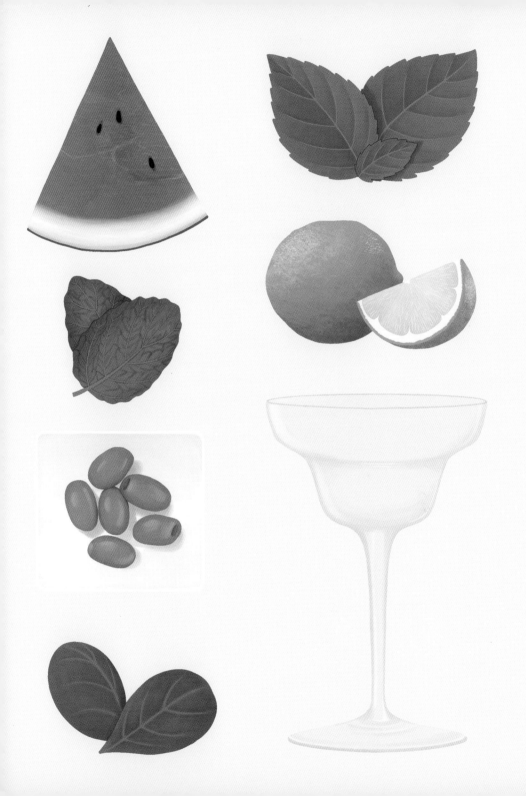

Shatavari Champagne Spritz

Inspired by the classic cocktail, the French 75, a celebratory champagne-based spritz, this sparkling aperitif is the perfect antidote to the lunchtime slump. The champagne vinegar and lemon oil alone help promote proper digestion. Add in shatavari, which is well known for promoting gut health, and goji berry juice for energy (not to mention it's bright pink hue and tart flavor), and this may just become your go-to adaptogenic beverage for all occasions.

The lemon oil in this recipe is extracted by macerating lemon peels with cane sugar. In the bar world, the resulting syrup is called *oleo saccharum,* a Latin phrase that translates to "sugary oil." Oleo saccharum is an ingredient that started popping up around the nineteenth century in cocktails, as a way of imparting citrus to a drink. It's stable and doesn't ferment like lemon juice does, which makes it one handy beverage ingredient to have around. In this recipe, I add champagne vinegar, turning it into more a shrub.

You can easily multiply this recipe for gatherings and brunches. It makes a great replacement for the basic mimosa, saving you a wicked hangover from cheap bubbly.

FOR THE GOJI BERRY JUICE

1 cup (106 g) goji berries

3 cups (24 oz or 710 ml) filtered water, plus more for soaking

FOR THE CHAMPAGNE OLEO SACCHRUM

1 cup (96 g) lemon peels

1 cup (200 g) cane sugar

2 ounces (60 ml) good-quality champagne vinegar

continued on next page

YIELD: 1 SPRITZ

TO MAKE THE GOJI BERRY JUICE: Add the goji berries to a bowl and cover completely with filtered water. Let the berries soak overnight to fully hydrate. When you're ready to make the juice, strain out the water the berries have been soaking in. Add the soaked berries and 3 cups (24 oz or 710 ml) of fresh filtered water to your blender. Blend on high for about 30 seconds. Strain through a fine-mesh strainer to remove the pulp, if desired. Store in an airtight container in the fridge for up to 5 days.

continued on next page

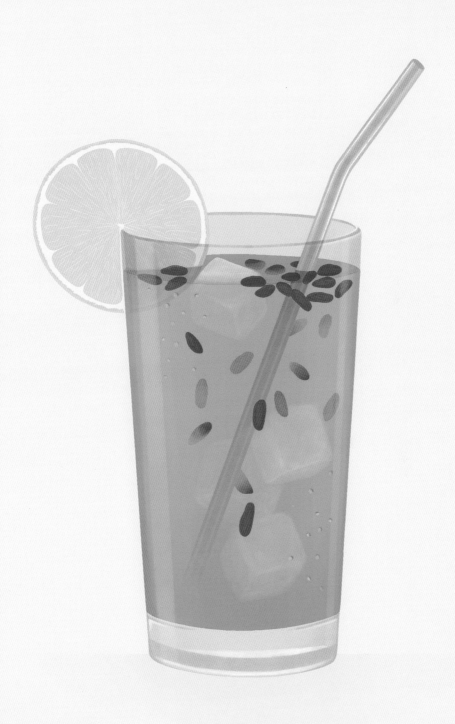

FOR THE SHATAVARI CHAMPAGNE SPRITZ

0.7 milliliter (14 drops) shatavari extract

3 ounces (90 ml) Goji Berry Juice or nectar

1 ounce (30 ml) Champagne Oleo Saccharum

1 ounce (30 ml) fresh-squeezed lemon juice

1 drop real vanilla extract

FOR SERVING

2 ounces (60 ml) limoncello La Croix or sparkling water of your choice

Lemon twist, for garnish

TO MAKE THE CHAMPAGNE OLEO SACCHARUM: Add the lemon peels and sugar to a sturdy bowl. Use your fingers to toss the sugar and peel together so the peels get nicely coated. Using a muddler or a wooden spoon, firmly press the lemon peels and sugar together until the peels start to express their oil. Cover the bowl with a cloth and let sit for at least 1 hour or up to a day. Once ready, strain the peels to separate the oil. Discard or set aside the peels; they can be used to flavor iced teas and lemonades if you wish. Stir the champagne vinegar into the oil. Store in an airtight container until ready to use.

TO MAKE THE SHATAVARI CHAMPAGNE SPRITZ: Add all the ingredients to your cocktail shaker or mason jar with a lid. Add 4 to 5 ice cubes and shake hard for 5 seconds.

TO SERVE: Pour the sparkling water into the shaker or jar. Strain into a chilled highball or coupe glass and garnish with a lemon twist.

PRO TIP
When peeling the lemons for the oleo saccharum, I use a Y-peeler to strip the peel without taking off the bitter white pith.

Hocus Focus Shot

The perfect antidote to afternoon brain drain is a dose of pine pollen, with its ability to support focus. Paired here with holy basil, which provides an instant mood boost, this powerful duo gets to work quickly, staving off that 3 p.m. slump when all you want to do is crawl under your desk for a catnap.

FOR THE CINNAMON SIMPLE SYRUP

1 cup (200 g) cane sugar

1 cup (8 oz or 235 ml) boiling water

4 whole cinnamon sticks

FOR THE HOCUS FOCUS SHOT

0.7 milliliter (14 drops) pine pollen extract

0.7 milliliter (14 drops) holy basil tincture

1 ounce (30 ml) chilled hibiscus tea

½ ounce (15 ml) Cinnamon Simple Syrup

YIELD: 1 SHOT

TO MAKE THE CINNAMON SIMPLE SYRUP: Add the sugar to a heatproof glass or bowl. Pour the boiling water over top and stir until the sugar dissolves. Add the cinnamon sticks to the warm syrup. Allow to steep for at least 24 hours in an airtight container in the fridge. I often leave the cinnamon sticks in the syrup even after I've started using it—the longer it rests in the syrup, the fuller the flavor.

TO MAKE THE HOCUS FOCUS SHOT: Add all the ingredients to your cocktail shaker or mason jar with a lid. Shake hard for about 5 seconds. Pour into a glass of your choice and drink immediately.

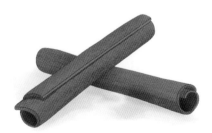

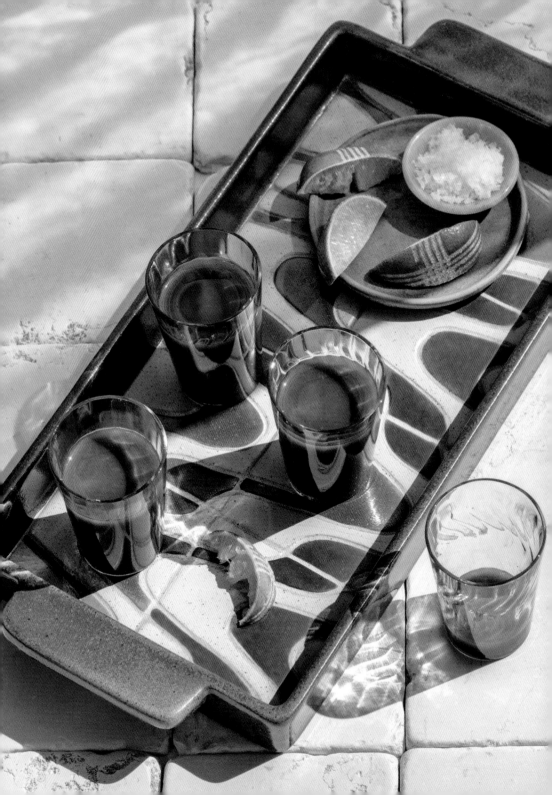

Glow Up! Shot

One of my favorite ways to cool down on a hot day is to make cucumber lemonade. The cucumber juice is just so cooling and refreshing! I mix batches of this up for gatherings as well as for afternoon glow shots, but however much you make, it's important that you drink it on the same day you juice the cucumbers. Cucumber juice can ferment quite quickly and turn sour, so make sure it's always fresh when you're drinking it.

I pair the cucumber lemonade with another cool cat, the skin-soothing aloe juice, which is also excellent for digestion and inflammation, as well as spirulina, for its nutritional density. But the star of this serotonin-booster is amla, for its mood-stabilizing and glow-conjuring abilities. You simply can't help but be in a good mood when you see what amla and her crew can do for you!

FOR THE GLOW UP! SHOT

½ teaspoon amla powder

1 teaspoon spirulina powder (see Notes)

1 ounce (30 ml) cucumber juice

½ ounce (15 ml) aloe vera juice

½ ounce (15 ml) fresh-squeezed lime juice

½ ounce (15 ml) honey syrup (see Notes)

FOR SERVING

Lime wedge

Sea salt

YIELD: 1 SHOT

TO MAKE THE GLOW UP! SHOT: Add all the ingredients to your blender and blend on high. Alternatively, add the ingredients to a small pitcher and whip using a milk frother. Pour into a glass and shoot.

TO SERVE: When I make this for friends, we typically shoot it like a tequila shot with limes and sea salt for a touch of festive fun.

NOTES

Spirulina is typically green, but blue majik spirulina from a region of the Pacific Northwest can also be found at higher-end health food stores. Either kind is fine in this recipe.

To make the honey syrup, mix equal parts honey with hot water and stir until the honey fully dissolves. Chill before using.

Elderberry Shrub Shot

Just because it's summer and it's sunny doesn't mean you're immune to getting run down and catching a cold. Some of my worst colds have happened as the summer starts to wind down and we head to that in-between time when the weather is on the verge of changing.

For this shrub-based immunity shot, I blend together elderberry extract, with its immune-boosting superpowers, and the last of the juicy summer blackberries from the market with ginger root, honey, and apple cider vinegar. The vinegar and honey work to extract the juices from the ripe berries and preserve them, preventing them from fermenting into blackberry wine. Keep a jar of this handy in your fridge and reach for it every time you start to feel run down and in need of a gingery hug.

0.7 milliliter (14 drops) black elderberry extract (see Notes)

1 cup (150 g) fresh ripe blackberries (see Notes)

1 cup (8 oz or 235 ml) runny honey

4 ounces (120 ml) apple cider vinegar

1 tablespoon (6 g) grated fresh ginger root

1 teaspoon grated lemon zest

YIELD: ABOUT 10 SHOTS

Add all the ingredients to a mason jar with a lid. Muddle the berries, ginger root, and lemon zest into the liquid and stir. Cover and store in the fridge in an airtight jar for at least 2 days to let the juice extract. When ready to drink, pour a small amount in the glass of your choosing and enjoy.

NOTES

Frozen berries work too, but because they've been frozen, there will be a certain amount of extra water in them from the ice so they're not as flavorful.

When purchasing elderberry extract, make sure you are purchasing the extract (it usually comes in a small dropper bottle), not elderberry syrup, which usually comes in a larger bottle and contains other ingredients.

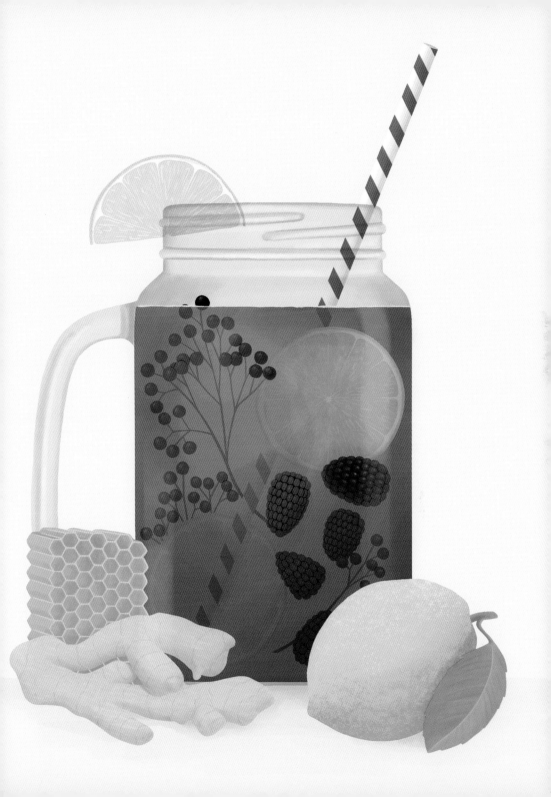

Goji Berry Go-Go Shot

This adaptogenic summer shot is perfect for those days when you're out about town and in need of an energy boost. Coconut water replenishes valuable electrolytes on a hot summer day, goji berries boost your energy, and rhodiola promotes endurance. If you like, feel free to multiply the ratios below to make extra of this invigorating drink, so your boots can keep on walking all day long.

FOR THE GOJI BERRY JUICE

1 cup (106 g) goji berries

3 cups (24 oz or 710 ml) filtered water, plus more for soaking

FOR THE GOJI BERRY GO-GO SHOT

1 ounce (30 ml) chilled Goji Berry Juice or nectar

0.7 milliliter (14 drops) rhodiola extract

2 ounces (60 ml) chilled virgin coconut water

YIELD: 1 SHOT

TO MAKE THE GOJI BERRY JUICE: Add the goji berries to a bowl and cover completely with filtered water. Let the berries soak overnight to fully hydrate. When you're ready to make the juice, strain out the water the berries have been soaking in. Add the soaked berries and 3 cups (24 oz or 710 ml) of filtered water to your blender. Blend on high for about 30 seconds. Strain through a fine-mesh strainer to remove the pulp, if desired. Store in an airtight container in the fridge for up to 5 days.

TO MAKE THE GOJI BERRY GO-GO SHOT: Pour all the ingredients into your mini thermos flask and shake together.

Frosé All Day

Since this is summer, I couldn't miss out on doing an adaptogenic take on one of the most popular beverages of the last few years, frosé, which is, at its simplest, a bottle of rosé that's been frozen with some additional flavorings such as sugar and lemon.

For this nonalcoholic frosé, I've included sea buckthorn and albizia, the former for its immunity and heart health–boosting properties and the latter for its ability to quiet the mind, encourage rest, and effect a peaceful sleep.

The recipe makes enough frosé cubes for four servings, but my recommendation for hot summer nights is to keep a few trays of these on hand in your freezer, so you can keep heatwaves at bay and have frosé all day, every day!

4 ounces (120 ml) water

½ cup (100 g) cane sugar

1 cup (125 g) fresh raspberries

4 teaspoons (20 g) sea buckthorn powder

2.8 milliliters (56 drops) albizia extract

1¾ cups (14 oz or 425 ml) white verjus

1¾ cups (14 oz or 425 ml) nonalcoholic pink gin

1 ounce (30 ml) nonalcoholic lemon bitters

YIELD: 4 SERVINGS

In a heavy-bottomed saucepan, add the water and sugar and stir over low heat until the sugar dissolves. Add the fresh raspberries and stir. Remove the pan from the heat and allow the raspberries to almost dissolve in the warm syrup. This will take around 15 minutes.

Carefully strain the pink syrup through a fine-mesh strainer, making sure not to push any seeds though the strainer.

Add the raspberry syrup and the remaining ingredients to your blender. Blitz for about 30 seconds. Pour the liquid into ice cube trays and freeze overnight.

TO SERVE: Remove the ice cubes, add them to your blender on the ice setting, and blend on high. If more liquid is needed to help crush the cubes, add a couple more ounces of nonalcoholic pink gin. Pour the frosé into chilled coupe or martini glasses and enjoy.

PRO TIP

Buying fresh raspberries can get expensive if you're making large batches of this recipe. For a cost-effective option, use a framboise raspberry syrup or plain raspberry syrup instead. Both are easy to find online.

Moroccan Mint Holy Basil Julep

Moroccan mint tea on its own already offers many health benefits: it's anti-inflammatory, helps with allergies, aids digestion, and calms stomach ulcers. It's delicious by itself, but also fantastic when used in a cocktail, and I've long used it in my riff on that summer staple, the mint julep.

For this version of the classic cocktail (or NO-cktail, rather, because it's booze-free), I've added burdock root and holy basil. Burdock adds to the digestive properties of the mint tea, while holy basil brings in good times and great vibes. Because this is a nightcap, I suggest making a weaker infusion of tea so that you have more of a gentle buzz.

FOR THE MOROCCAN MINT TEA

1 teaspoon (4 g) gunpowder green tea pearls

½ cup (48 g) fresh spearmint leaves (Do not include stems.)

2 cups (16 oz or 475 ml) boiling hot water

FOR THE STRAWBERRY ROSE SYRUP

½ cup (113 g) fresh ripe strawberries, leaves removed

1 cup (8 oz or 235 ml) chilled simple syrup (see Pro Tips)

1 ounce (30 ml) rose water, such as Al Wadi brand

YIELD: 1 JULEP

TO MAKE THE MOROCCAN MINT TEA: Add the tea and mint leaves into a tea-infusing vessel of your choice. Pour over the boiling water and allow to steep for about 15 minutes or up to 1 hour. Remove the tea and mint leaves and chill before using.

TO MAKE THE STRAWBERRY ROSE SYRUP: Add all the ingredients to your blender and blitz on high for about 30 seconds. Strain the syrup through a fine-mesh strainer, pushing it through with a wooden spoon and making sure not to push any seeds though the strainer. Store in an airtight container in the fridge for up to 5 days.

TO MAKE THE MOROCCAN MINT HOLY BASIL JULEP: In a chilled glass or julep cup, add the mint leaves and syrup and muddle lightly. You don't want to crush the leaves completely, just release some of their oils. Add the burdock and holy basil extracts and fill the glass halfway with crushed ice. Pour in the chilled tea and swirl or swizzle the drink with a long spoon (see Pro Tips). Top with more crushed ice and garnish with a bushy mint sprig.

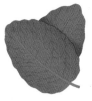

FOR THE MOROCCAN MINT HOLY BASIL JULEP

6 fresh mint leaves

1 ounce (30 ml) Strawberry Rose Syrup

2 milliliters (40 drops) burdock root extract

0.7 milliliter (14 drops) holy basil extract

4 ounces (120 ml) chilled Moroccan Mint Tea

Bushy mint sprig, for garnish

PRO TIPS

Swizzling is a technique used in cocktails that contain crushed ice, with the spoon (or swizzle stick) acting like a blender. To swizzle a drink, place the bowl of the spoon into the glass of ice and place the handle between the flat palms of your hands. Rub your palms together, twirling the spoon handle as if you were making fire. This works best when you have only a half-filled glass of ice; if its full, the ice will swizzle on out of the glass and end up all over the floor.

Make the simple syrup for this recipe ahead of time. Mix equal parts cane sugar and hot water, stirring until the sugar dissolves completely. Allow to cool before using, and refrigerate it to store.

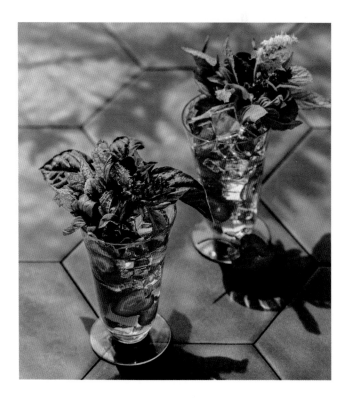

Turmeric Maca Paleta

Ice cream is one of the best things about summer—except that it's packed with so much sugar! During the pandemic, I spent months trying to make delicious low-sugar ice creams, freezer pops, and paletas. The paleta, a traditional Mexican frozen treat, quickly became my favorite because it's easy to make, packed with flavor, doesn't require too many fancy tools, and freezes relatively quickly.

For this adaptogenic paleta, I added maca and turmeric, both for their mood-enhancing and immune-boosting properties. The rest of the flavor profile is inspired by Thai ingredients: makrut lime leaf for its floral qualities, and coconut and ginger root to complement the turmeric.

4½ ounces (134 ml) full-fat coconut milk

10 makrut lime leaves

4 teaspoons (20 g) maca powder

1 ounce (28 g) fresh turmeric root, peeled

2 ounces (56 g) fresh ginger root, peeled

¾ cup (57 g) unsweetened coconut flakes

5 ounces (150 ml) sweetened condensed coconut milk or regular condensed milk

Pinch of sea salt

1 ounce (28 g) black sesame seeds

YIELD: 4 SERVINGS

In a heavy-bottomed saucepan, add the coconut milk and makrut lime leaves. Bring to a simmer over medium heat. Turn the heat off and let the makrut limes leaves steep in the coconut milk for up to 8 hours. The longer they steep, the more flavor you'll get.

Once the coconut milk is infused to your satisfaction and cooled to room temperature, remove the lime leaves and pour the infused milk into your blender. Add all the remaining ingredients, except the sesame seeds, and blend on high until smooth. Stir in the sesame seeds.

Pour the paleta custard into metal popsicle molds; metal helps the custard freeze faster. Place the lids on the molds and insert popsicle sticks so that only a third of the stick is visible. Freeze for about 6 hours or overnight. (If you can wait that long!)

To remove the paletas, place the filled molds in warm water one at a time. This should loosen the paletas and make them easy to pull out. At this point, either put them back in the freezer as is or, for a sweeter treat, dip them in melted chocolate and then in coconut flakes and/or black sesame seeds. When you are ready to re-freeze them, wrap them in parchment paper, place them on a freezer tray, and pop the tray back into the freezer until ready to eat.

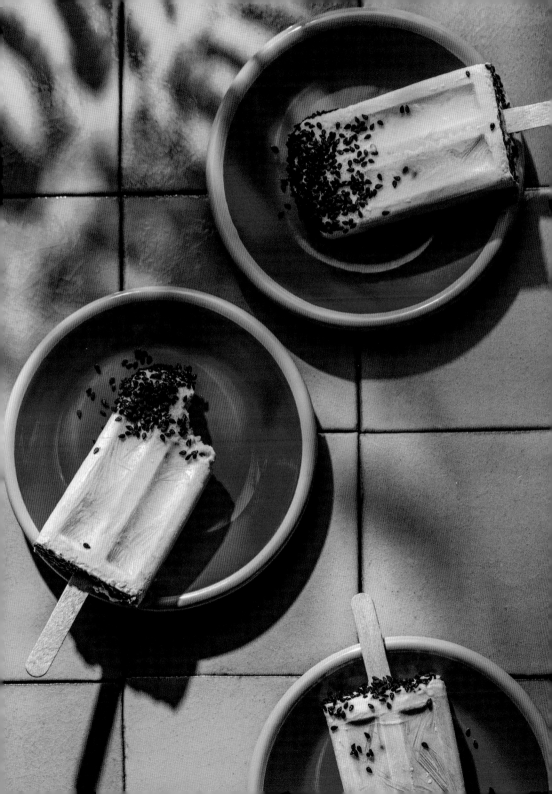

Eastern Crush

This adaptogenic nightcap is inspired by a classic Singapore sling, which features cherry liqueur quite heavily. My booze-free version relies on tart cherry juice, rumored to be an excellent sleep aid, and pineapple juice for its digestive qualities. To this I've added the wonder fungi reishi, used for centuries in Traditional Chinese Medicine to help with depression and anxiety, as well as for allergies and immunity.

The classic way to serve a sling is over rocks in a highball-style glass, but with my preference for ice-free beverages, I like to serve it up in a cocktail coupe. Of course, feel free to follow your own instincts here!

1 milliliter (20 drops) reishi tincture

1 ounce (30 ml) unsweetened tart cherry juice

1½ ounces (45 ml) unsweetened pineapple juice

½ ounce (15 ml) fresh-squeezed lemon juice

1 ounce (30 ml) simple syrup (see Note)

3 dashes nonalcoholic orange bitters

1 drop real vanilla extract

Skewered cherry, for garnish

YIELD: 1 DRINK

Add all the ingredients with 4 ice cubes to your cocktail shaker or mason jar with a lid. Shake hard for 5 seconds. Strain into a chilled cocktail coupe glass. Garnish with a cherry on a skewer.

NOTE

Make the simple syrup for this recipe ahead of time. Mix equal parts cane sugar and hot water, stirring until the sugar dissolves completely. Allow to cool before using, and refrigerate it to store.

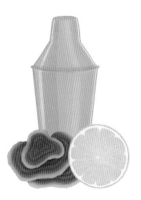

Fuzzy Navel Punch with Rhodiola

Back in the '80s, the Fuzzy Navel was a popular cocktail made of a simple combination of peach schnapps and orange juice (fuzzy—peach, navel—orange). Sometimes a shot of vodka was added if you wanted a quicker buzz. For this recipe, I replace the alcohol with adaptogenic powerhouses rhodiola and goji berry. Both these adaptogens bring their wealth of superhero, fatigue-fighting talents to this mix, with rhodiola giving the left hook to anxiety and depression, knocking it way out the door.

For me, peaches are always associated with mint and sweet iced tea. In this recipe, however, I suggest using rooibos or red bush tea rather than standard black tea; its subtle sweet woody notes are a great complement to juicy ripe peaches. And because this is a drink for parties, I top it off with a nonalcoholic sparkling wine such as Le Blanc from French Bloom. If you want something a bit more casual, sparkling elderflower lemonade can give this punch bowl a touch of effervescence to fizz up your night.

FOR THE FUZZY NAVEL PUNCH WITH RHODIOLA

1¼ teaspoons (120 drops or 6 ml) rhodiola extract

1 cup (8 oz or 235 ml) chilled Goji Berry Juice (page 55) or nectar

2 cups (16 oz or 475 ml) chilled rooibos tea

2 cups (16 oz or 475 ml) chilled peach nectar or puree

4 ounces (120 ml) fresh-squeezed lemon juice

4 ounces (120 ml) chilled simple syrup (see Note, page 34)

2 cups (16 oz or 475 ml) chilled nonalcoholic champagne or sparkling lemonade

FOR SERVING

Bushy mint sprigs, for garnish

YIELD: 8 SERVINGS

TO MAKE THE FUZZY NAVEL PUNCH WITH RHODIOLA: Add all the ingredients to a pitcher and stir together. Add ice cubes or ring mold ice (see Pro Tip for directions) to your punch bowl and pour punch over top. Add some lemon or peach slices to the bowl as decoration.

TO SERVE: Ladle into punch glasses and garnish with a bushy mint sprig.

PRO TIP

I love making ring mold ice for this recipe; it adds a wonderful fancy touch! Simply pour water into a babka ring mold and add lemon slices. Freeze overnight and dunk into warm water when ready to release the ice from the mold. Place the ring mold ice into your punch bowl with the curved side of the ice mold facing upward.

Sandíalada

Next to the holidays, summertime is the best time of year for get-togethers, from picnics in the park to lazy Sundays at the beach to barbecues in the backyard. The ubiquitous summer beverage for many at such gatherings is an ice-cold beer. The problem with that, of course, is that within a few minutes of drinking one, your body starts to dehydrate, thanks to alcohol's diuretic properties.

I've mentioned in previous recipes that the availability of excellent nonalcoholic beers has proliferated in the last few years, with some of the best brew houses jumping onto the NA trend. Like any good Englishwoman, my favorite way of drinking these delicious beverages is by mixing them with lemonade to make a shandy. In Mexico, they have a similar drink: the michelada, an ice-cold ale mixed with lime juice, hot sauce, and salt. The michelada forms the basis of this recipe, but I take it a step further by adding watermelon, the ultimate summer fruit, to make what I call a sandíalada (*sandía* being the name for watermelon in Spanish).

For my adaptogenic ingredients, I like to add shatavari to this elixir because of its fantastic fatigue-fighting powers. I also include moringa, for its ability to relieve anxiety, lower blood pressure, and aid digestion. All of that can come in handy come party time, especially if you're hosting or if you have a sensitive tummy that might not do so well with indulgent summer party food.

Make sure this one gets enjoyed quickly—the last thing you want at your party is flat beer!

FOR THE SANDÍALADA

1¼ teaspoons (120 drops or 6 ml) moringa extract

1 scant teaspoon (90 drops or 4.5 ml) shatavari extract

2¼ cups (18 oz or 540 ml) fresh ripe watermelon juice

3 ounces (90 ml) fresh-squeezed lime juice

1 to 2 ounces (30 to 60 ml) hot sauce

FOR SERVING

3 cups (24 oz or 710 ml) chilled nonalcoholic pilsner or wheat beer

Lime wedges

Sea salt or Tajín, for the rim

Watermelon wedges

YIELD: 6 TO 8 SERVINGS

TO MAKE THE SANDÍALADA: Add all the ingredients to a chilled pitcher and stir. Store in the fridge until you're ready to serve—you want to add the beer just before serving so it doesn't go flat.

TO SERVE: Pour in the NA beer. Rub a lime wedge around the rim of your chilled glasses and dip them in sea salt or Tajín. Fill the glasses with ice and pour in the sandíalada. Garnish with a watermelon or lime wedge.

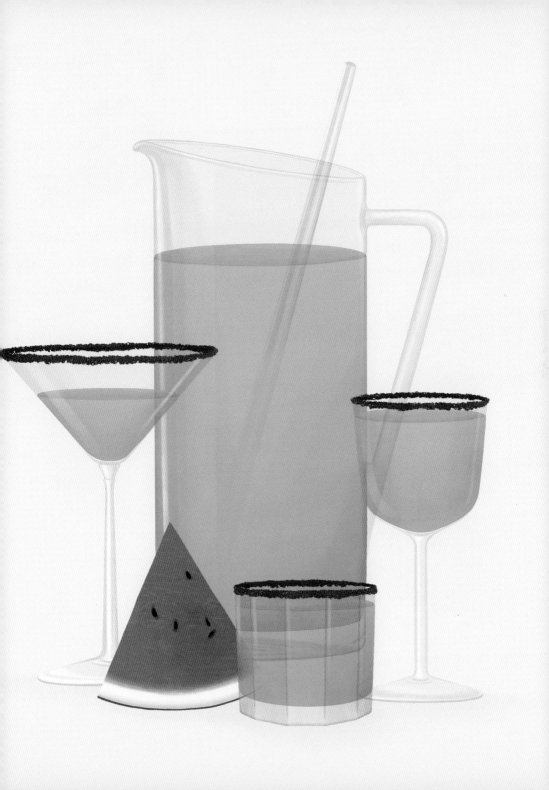

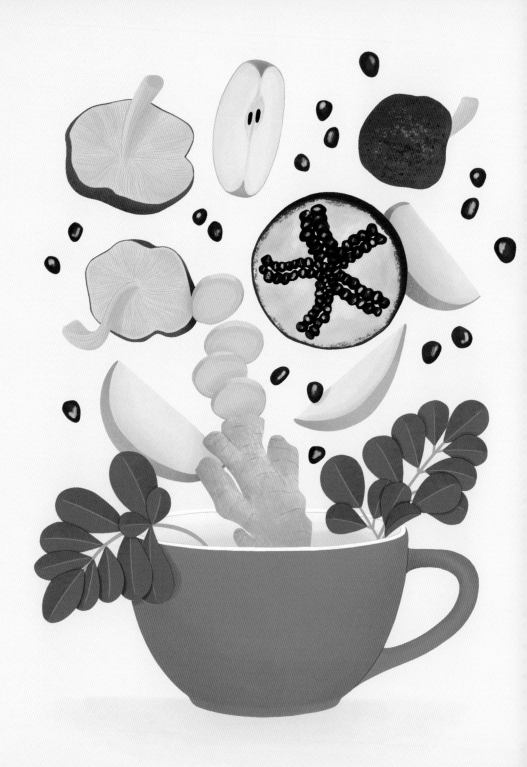

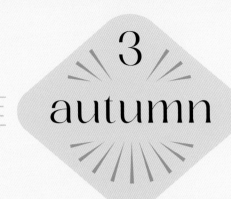

3
autumn

After the joy of long summer days, bare feet, and all that sweet sunshine, shifting into autumn gear can sometimes bring about the blues. At least, this is true for me. To counteract this seasonal sadness, I make sure that I stock up on a plethora of adaptogens, with their abundance of neuro-assisting phytochemical magic: rhodiola, ashwagandha, licorice, maca, holy basil. Adaptogenic culinary ingredients such as shiitake mushrooms and turmeric also become more frequent additions to my cooking escapades during this time of year.

However, for many, this is a season for fulfillment. In countries such as Denmark and Sweden, instead of lamenting this shift, they lean into this time of year and celebrate it with *hygge*. The word dates to the 1800s and describes a mood of slowing down and spending time in cozy conviviality—alone or with loved ones—to promote a sense of contentment and wellness. Hygge is all about bundling up and creating oases of calm and comfy tranquility, spending quiet time reading books by the fire, with warming drinks and soothing foods. It is a time to rest and reset.

The delicious beverages in this chapter are inspired by this attitude and feature an assortment of warming baking spices to help you cultivate this frame of mind. These pantry staples create that sense of comfort, as well as delivering a fix of polyphenols that have protective, antioxidant properties for your holistic health.

Orchard fruits such as apples, pears, and pomegranate proliferate in this chapter, as does ginger root and a few of my favorite tropical fruits that become abundant in the fall. A piña colada might seem like it's more suited to summer by the pool, but mix it with some aromatic spices and you have a delish holiday-inspired variation.

So if you're ready, might I suggest wrapping up in your favorite cozy woolly sweater or tucking up in a blanket and prepare to toast the season of hygge!

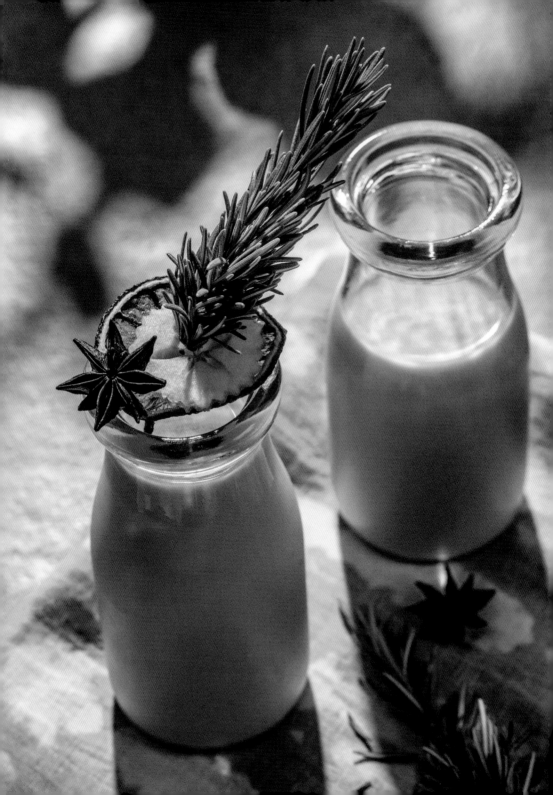

Apple Pine Pollen Shake

While apples may seem like an unassuming member of the fruit family, there is some credence to the adage, "An apple a day keeps the doctor away." Apples are packed full of healthful benefits: keeping teeth clean, helping with digestion and weight loss, decreasing the risk of diabetes, keeping the brain and heart healthy, and even helping to fight cancer. Apples also happen to be a rich source of that allergy-busting phytochemical, quercetin.

Adding to this bonanza of benefits, the adaptogens pine pollen and schisandra berry bring their brain-promoting, anxiety-fighting, and immune-boosting properties to the mix. Pine pollen also helps with energy while schisandra berry assists with endurance.

The recipe is based on an apple-buttermilk nitrogen-frozen slushy I used to make at one of my fancy restaurants many moons ago. Laced with seasonal mulling spices, it's the perfect sipper to put you in that autumnal, "holidays are on the way!" mood. The icy element here comes from frozen bananas, which also provide bulk to this delightful morning shake. It will quickly become your favorite way to keep that proverbial doctor at bay!

1 heaped teaspoon (5 g) pine pollen powder

2 milliliters (40 drops) schisandra berry extract

1 fruity apple, cored and sliced

1 frozen banana

4 ounces (120 ml) fresh-pressed apple cider

2 ounces (60 ml) cashew nut milk

¼ teaspoon grated lemon zest

¼ teaspoon ground cinnamon

¼ teaspoon freshly grated nutmeg

¼ teaspoon ground allspice

½ teaspoon ground ginger

Pinch of sea salt

YIELD: 1 SHAKE

Add all the ingredients to your blender and blend on high until smooth.

Mango Maca Lassi

Originating in India, a classic lassi is a cooling yogurt-based drink that is said to have Ayurvedic healing properties because of the spices, such as cardamom and cumin, that are whipped into it. It's made with yogurt and naturally contains an abundance of vitamins and nutrients too, such as vitamin B, calcium, and folic acid. In this recipe, I've added maca, for its mood-enhancing, immune-boosting magic, and Siberian ginseng to wake up those brain cells and help with endurance. The icing on the cake here is fresh, or pureed, mango and cardamom, both packed full of antioxidants that can help with digestion and support healthy skin and hair.

If you're lucky enough to find Alphonso mangos, which are only available from around May to June, I highly recommend stocking up on this most exquisite and fragrant of varietals. They freeze beautifully and can carry you through the colder winter seasons, bringing a burst of intoxicating sunshine to your mornings. If you happen to live near an Indian or Southeast Asian supermarket, you can also find canned mango puree, an excellent substitute, which also makes an incredible mango limeade.

The consistency of this drink is similar to a smoothie, and it's an easy, incredibly delicious way to start your day, especially if you're someone who is always on the run in the morning, rushing to get to work or school. It will provide the energy you need to get out the door without making you feel sluggish. And if you've got time, it can be used as a basis for an acai bowl that can be layered with granola, nuts, bananas, and coconut.

2.8 milliliters (56 drops) maca tincture or 4 teaspoons (20 g) maca powder

2.8 milliliters (56 drops) Siberian ginseng tincture

3 cups (525 g) chopped mango or 2 cups (16 oz or 475 ml) mango puree

2 cups (16 oz or 475 ml) plain, unsweetened dairy or plant-based yogurt of your choice

1 cup (8 oz or 235 ml) virgin coconut water or full-fat coconut milk

2 tablespoons (30 ml) runny honey (optional)

Zest of 1 lime

1 teaspoon ground cardamom

4 drops real vanilla extract

½ teaspoon sea salt (optional)

½ teaspoon freshly grated nutmeg, for serving

YIELD: 4 SERVINGS

Add all the ingredients to your blender and blend on high for 30 seconds. Pour into chilled glass or to-go cup, and sprinkle with freshly grated nutmeg.

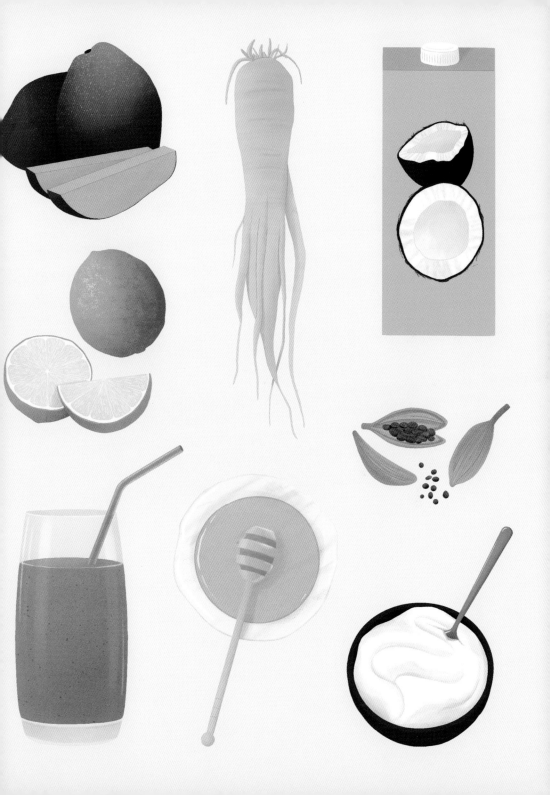

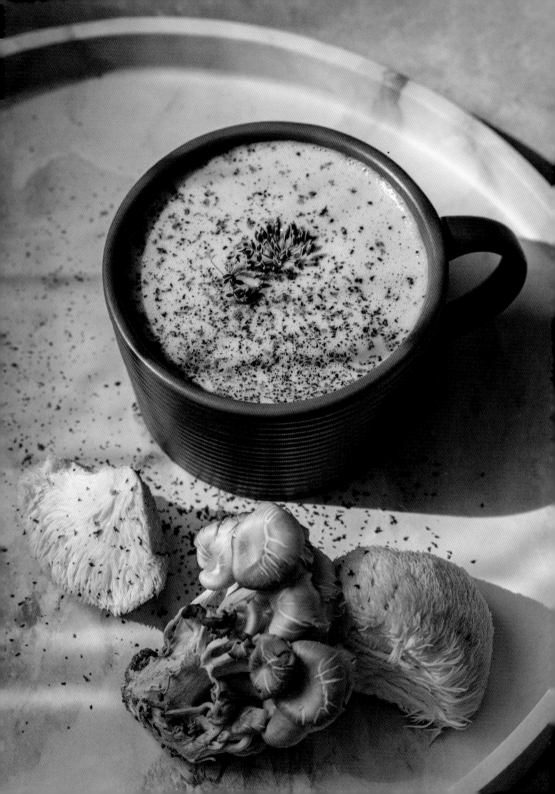

Dirty Chaga Chai

My favorite hygge-inspired morning beverage is, of course, hot chocolate. Since I started mixing drinks, I've always looked for ways to revamp classics and make them unique in some way. Hot chocolate goes so well with cinnamon, so why not chai? In barista terminology, a dirty chai refers to chai tea laced with a shot of espresso. While this is quite delicious, in this recipe, I use chocolate to make the drink "dirty." Both dark chocolate and chai spices bring a mix of potent polyphenols to this morning time treat, but add a dose of that king of all mushrooms, chaga, to the mix and you've got a fantastic way to start your day.

The adaptogen chaga has been used for centuries, especially in northern European countries, to treat many ailments including cancer. In preclinical studies carried out at the Memorial Sloan Kettering Cancer Center, this fantastic fungus showed antitumor, antiviral, antioxidant, anti-inflammatory, analgesic, antiallergic and cognition-enhancing properties. It's no wonder it's suddenly become so popular!

This recipe is not something to whip up when you're in a rush, as the chai takes some time to properly steep in the warm milk. I recommend saving this for a lazy weekend morning to enjoy with your Sunday paper in bed. Bonus: The infused milk will keep in the fridge for a couple days, so make extra to enjoy a dirty chaga chai several days in a row!

FOR THE DIRTY CHAGA CHAI

1 cup (8 oz or 235 ml) dairy or plant-based milk of your choice

1 black, green, or rooibos chai tea bag

½ teaspoon ground ginger

¼ teaspoon ground turmeric

Pinch of sea salt

1 teaspoon runny honey (optional)

1 ounce (28 g) dark chocolate

1 teaspoon chaga mushroom powder

1 drop real vanilla extract

FOR SERVING

Ground cinnamon

Shaved chocolate

YIELD: 1 CHAI LATTE

TO MAKE THE DIRTY CHAGA CHAI: Add the milk and tea bag to a small heavy-bottomed saucepan, and allow it to steep over very low heat for about 10 minutes. Remove the pan from the heat and let the tea bag sit for another 10 minutes. Remove the tea bag and squeeze between two teaspoons into the saucepan. Place the saucepan back over low heat and add the spices, salt, runny honey (if using), and chocolate, stirring until the chocolate fully dissolves. Add the chaga and vanilla. Blend everything together with a milk frother or stick blender.

TO SERVE: Transfer to a mug of your choice, and sprinkle some cinnamon and shaved chocolate over the top.

Mushroom Morning Glory Latte

If you're on social media these days, you've probably noticed all the ads for mushroom coffee that have been popping up recently. But when you click these links and read through the blurb, you discover not only the benefits of mushroom coffee but also how expensive some of these products are! Fortunately, it's easy to make a mushroom coffee at home for just a fraction of this cost by picking up shiitake powder, which, most of the time, costs under $20 and yields about 250 servings.

I chose shiitake mushrooms as my adaptogen here, because like chaga, they have a myriad of benefits. Most especially, they are fantastic for immune health, energy, and virility. Add a touch of reishi to this cuppa love, as well as a reviving spritz of orange oil, and you will feel like the king of the world.

FOR THE MUSHROOM MORNING GLORY LATTE

½ teaspoon shiitake mushroom powder

1 milliliter (20 drops) reishi extract

1 cup (8 oz or 235 ml) dairy or plant-based milk of your choice

½ ounce (15 ml) espresso or ½ teaspoon espresso powder

¼ teaspoon ground cinnamon

¼ teaspoon ground cardamom

Pinch of sea salt

FOR SERVING

Orange peel, for oil spritzing

YIELD: 1 LATTE

TO MAKE THE MUSHROOM MORNING GLORY LATTE: Add all the ingredients to a small heavy-bottomed saucepan over low heat and allow to heat through, approximately 3 minutes. Do not let the mixture come to boil, because you will burn the milk. Once the mixture has almost reached a low simmer, turn off the heat and whisk with a milk frother until the powders are well incorporated.

TO SERVE: Transfer the latte to a warm mug and spritz the orange oil from the peel over your latte by pinching it over the mug.

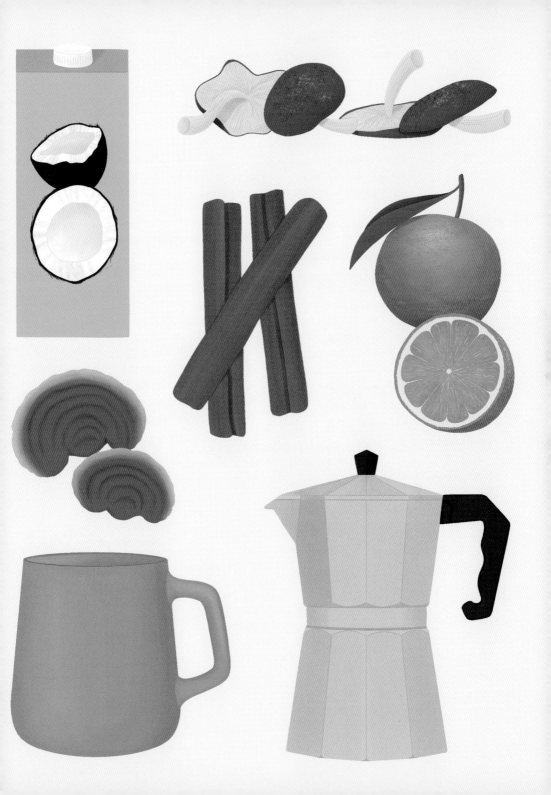

PPP Moringa Spritz

This recipe is an autumnal favorite of mine. I love its beautiful purple hue, baking spice aromas, and rich fruit-forward flavors. The base of this aperitif is a punch-like infusion called chicha morada. Chicha morada originated in the Andean mountains and is made by infusing dried purple corn, which you can find in Latin American markets or online, and apples, pineapple, cinnamon, and sometimes cloves or ginger root. Purple corn, or *maíz morado* as it's called in Peru, is rich in antioxidants and phytonutrients, particularly anthocyanin, which is a potent anti-inflammatory, as well as being an anticarcinogenic, aiding cardiovascular health, and fighting diabetes. You can see why I love this ingredient!

The punch takes some time to prepare: I recommend making this on a weekend or setting it up on the stove after dinner so it can steep overnight. The longer it steeps, the fuller the flavors will be. Once the infusion is fully steeped and chilled, this delightful spritz comes together very quickly and requires just three ingredients.

As for moringa, our protagonist in this Peruvian Purple Punch (PPP), it functions mainly as an antianxiety supplement; however, it's also incredibly beneficial for digestion, blood pressure, and antiaging. I've also added goji berries to the infusion for their energy kick for those of you who, like me, are always on the run.

FOR THE CHICHA MORADO

1 pound (454 g) dried purple corn

½ pineapple, peel included, chopped into cubes

6 whole cinnamon sticks

1 teaspoon cloves

¼ cup (50 g) cane sugar

¼ cup (27 g) goji berries

¼ cup (60 g) peeled, chopped fresh ginger root (see Pro Tips)

2 quarts (1.9 L) fresh-pressed apple cider or juice

2 quarts (1.9 L) filtered water

1 to 2 ounces (30 to 60 ml) apple cider vinegar (optional)

YIELD: 1 SPRITZ

TO MAKE THE CHICHA MORADA: Add all the ingredients, except the apple cider vinegar, to a large, heavy-bottomed, lidded pan such as a cast-iron casserole dish. Place the dish on the stove over medium heat and bring to a simmer. Reduce the heat to low and cover with the lid. Allow it to stew for at least 2 hours.

Remove the chicha morado from the heat and chill in the fridge overnight or up to 12 hours.

Remove from the fridge and strain the liquid through a fine-mesh strainer to remove the solids. Add apple cider vinegar 1 ounce (30 ml) at a time (if using). Store in the fridge for about 1 week.

**FOR THE PPP
MORINGA SPRITZ**

3 ounces (90 ml) Chicha Morado

1 milliliter (20 drops)
moringa extract

2 to 3 ounces (60 to 90 ml)
sparkling nonalcoholic
apple cider

Orange twist, for garnish

TO MAKE THE PPP SPRITZ: Add the chicha morado, along with the moringa, to a highball or wine glass and top with ice. Pour in the nonalcoholic sparkling apple cider of your choice and garnish with a twist of orange.

PRO TIPS
To remove the skin from the ginger root, use the back of a teaspoon to scrape it away rather than peeling it with a knife. You'll retain so much more of the valuable root this way.

If you're a baker (like me!) and have any fruit scraps lying around such as apple peels or apple cores, you can add these to the infusion too. I try using every part of my fruit and veg (for stocks) so there's zero waste.

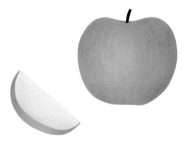

Vie En Rose "Margarita" with Holy Basil

Revered for its health benefits, the pomegranate contains about three times more anti-oxidants and phenols than green tea and red wine. It boosts heart and urinary health, and it aids in fighting stomach ailments, diabetes, and carcinogens. In studies over the last few decades, there is also evidence that pomegranates help reduce inflammation of all the organs.

To me, pomegranate is one of those flavors that signifies autumn and the approaching holidays. Rose and pistachio (in other words, the flavors of Turkish delight) are two others.

As it happens, pomegranates and rose water are a classic flavor pairing in the Middle East, particularly Syria. The beverage that follows is probably one of the most crushable and craveable nonalcoholic margarita-inspired recipes in my arsenal, and I have made many variations of it throughout my years as a mixologist.

To add to this heavenly combination, my adaptogenic supplements here are holy basil for its instant mood lift, plus rhodiola to fight the blues and promote mental clarity, as well as a boost of energy to ward off the afternoon slumps.

All in all, I hope my Vie en Rose "Margarita" truly encourages you to see life though rose-tinted glasses!

0.7 milliliter (14 drops) holy basil extract

0.7 milliliter (14 drops) rhodiola extract

2½ ounces (75 ml) fresh pomegranate juice

1 ounce (30 ml) fresh-squeezed lemon juice

½ ounce (15 ml) simple syrup (see Note)

¼ ounce (8 ml) rose water, such as Al Wadi brand

Pinch of sea salt

Rose petal, for garnish (optional)

YIELD: 1 "MARGARITA"

Add all the ingredients with 4 ice cubes to your cocktail shaker or mason jar with a lid. Shake hard for 5 seconds. Strain into a chilled glass filled with ice and garnish with a rose petal if you're feeling fancy.

NOTE
Make the simple syrup for this recipe ahead of time. Mix equal parts cane sugar and hot water, stirring until the sugar dissolves completely. Allow to cool before using, and refrigerate it to store.

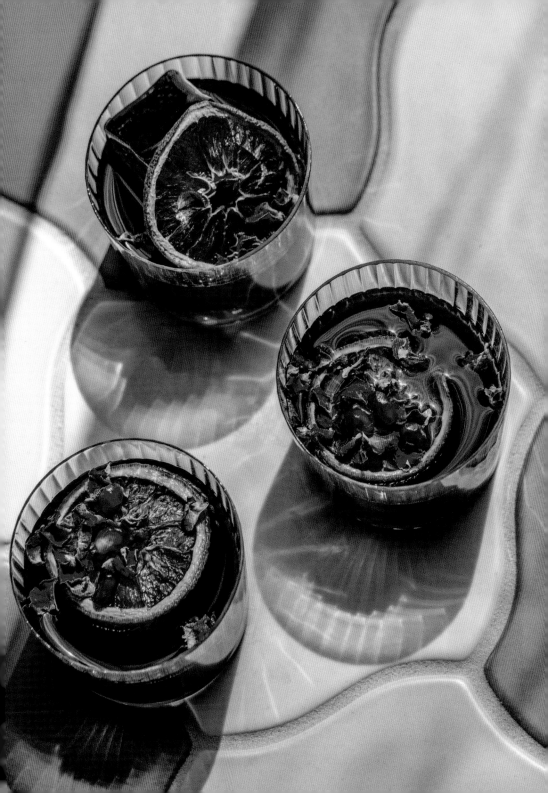

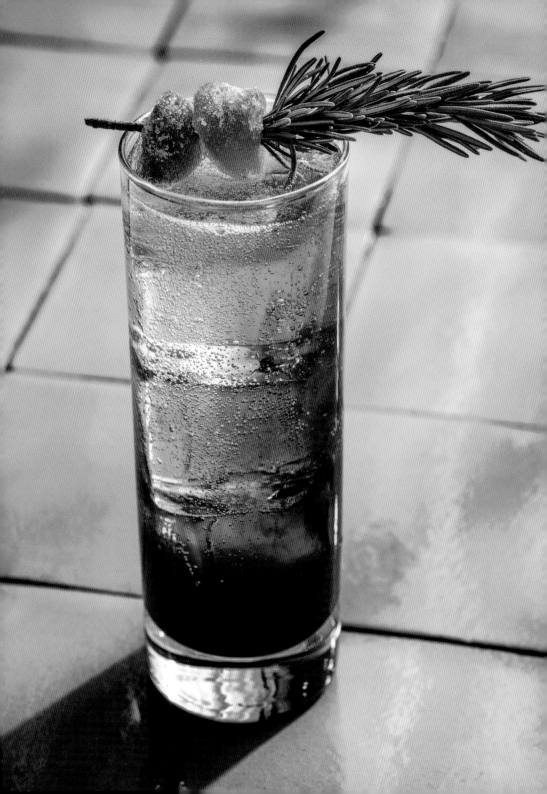

Elder Diablito

You've probably guessed that this recipe is inspired by the El Diablo, a cocktail traditionally composed of tequila, ginger, and crème de cassis. To make this version medicinal rather than indulgent, I replace the black currant flavor of crème de cassis with elderberry. Tart, juicy elderberries have been used for centuries in folk medicine to help ward off colds and treat sciatica, while in ancient Egypt it was used to heal burns and boost their complexions. These days, elderberries are one of the most commonly used plant medicines in the world. Because all the health-promoting ingredients make this alcohol-free drink hardly a devil, I like to use the diminutive diablito.

As for the adaptogen in this beneficial beverage, amla is employed to bring about a boost of energy and aid digestion, as well as being a powerful partner in banishing the blues.

FOR THE GINGER SYRUP

1 cup (240 g) peeled, chopped fresh ginger root

2 cups (400 g) cane sugar

2 cups (16 oz or 475 ml) hot water

FOR THE ELDER DIABLITO

0.7 milliliter (14 drops) amla tincture

0.7 milliliter (14 drops) black elderberry tincture

½ ounce (15 ml) elderberry liquid

2 ounces (60 ml) zero-proof tequila

¾ ounce (22 ml) Ginger Syrup

½ ounce (15 ml) fresh-squeezed lime juice

FOR SERVING

1 ounce (30 ml) ginger beer or club soda, for topping off

Candied ginger

YIELD: 1 DRINK

TO MAKE THE GINGER SYRUP: Blend all the ingredients together on high for about 30 seconds. Strain though a fine-mesh strainer, pushing the liquid through the solids with the back of a tablespoon or small ladle. Store in an airtight container in the fridge for up to 7 days.

TO MAKE THE ELDER DIABLITO: Add all the ingredients with 4 to 5 ice cubes to your cocktail shaker or mason jar with a lid. Shake hard for 5 seconds.

TO SERVE: Add a splash of ginger beer (about an ounce) or club soda to the shaker. Strain into a chilled highball glass filled with ice and garnish with candied ginger on a toothpick.

Astragalus Toffee Apple Sour

This sour provides a one-two punch of energy from adaptogens Siberian ginseng, which brings its powers of focus, endurance, and muscle-building, and astragalus, which confers its immune-boosting powers. Together these two supplements are a formidable ally in your fight to get through the cooler, darker months of the year.

While the lemon juice and apple cider vinegar do still render this drink a sour, I've downplayed the tanginess a little in this recipe by adding a touch of maple syrup to represent the classic candied apples often picked up at farmers' markets and fairs at this time of year.

FOR THE ASTRAGALUS TOFFEE APPLE SOUR

1 milliliter (20 drops) Siberian ginseng extract

2 milliliters (40 drops) astragalus root extract

2½ ounces (75 ml) fresh-pressed apple cider or juice

1 ounce (30 ml) fresh-squeezed lemon juice

½ ounce (15 ml) Grade-A Vermont maple syrup or caramel syrup

¼ ounce (8 ml) apple cider vinegar (optional)

1 ounce (30 ml) aquafaba or egg white (optional)

Pinch of ground cinnamon

FOR SERVING

Lemon twist, for oil spritzing

YIELD: 1 SOUR

TO MAKE THE ASTRAGALUS TOFFEE APPLE SOUR: Add all the ingredients with 1 ice cube to your cocktail shaker or mason jar with a lid. Shake hard for 10 seconds. Add 3 more ice cubes and shake again for 5 seconds.

TO SERVE: Strain immediately into a chilled coupe or stemmed glass of your choice. Finish with a spritz of lemon oil from a twist pinched over the glass.

PRO TIP

If you're feeling adventurous, try shaking this sour with the lemon peel inside the tin or mason jar. The drink get infused with the oils from the peel as the ice and shaking beats the lemon twist inside. This style of shaking is known in the professional bar world as a regal shake.

Turmeric Shatavari Zinger

This next recipe contains two ingredients that belong to the ginger family, turmeric and ginger, the roots of which are often used as culinary ingredients. Turmeric is a key player here, a powerful anti-inflammatory and antioxidant that has been used for centuries in Ayurveda and Traditional Chinese Medicine because of its high level of the polyphenol known as curcumin. Like many other colorful plant-based foods, turmeric is known to protect the body by fighting free radicals and shielding our cells from damage. It is an excellent adaptogen to take for help with arthritis and digestive ailments. It also aids cognitive functioning, is a powerful general immune booster and mood booster, and is purported to support a youthful glow.

To this warming, immune-boosting shot, I've also added ginger root and a dose of shatavari, to create a triple punch of cold and allergy-fighting power. Shatavari also delivers on the gut health front too. To round this all out, manuka honey and apple cider vinegar bring up the rear with their antimicrobial properties to make this an essential cold-fighting weapon to have in your arsenal.

1 milliliter (20 drops) turmeric extract

0.7 milliliter (14 drops) shatavari extract

½ ounce (15 ml) ginger juice

1 ounce (30 ml) homemade manuka honey syrup (see Note)

½ ounce (15 ml) apple cider vinegar

2 ounces (60 ml) hot water

YIELD: 1 SHOT

Add all the ingredients to a glass and stir or whisk with a milk frother wand. Drink immediately.

NOTE
Make manuka honey syrup at home by combining equal parts honey and warm water and mixing until the honey dissolves.

American Pie Shot

For this autumn-inspired brain-boosting shot, I decided to pair American ginseng with cranberry, that quintessential New England berry originally cultivated by the people of the Algonquian Nation. American ginseng is known for its ability to stimulate the central nervous system and improve cognitive functioning. It also boosts immunity and endurance, and is the perfect afternoon pick-me-up for when your energy starts to wane. As for the humble cranberry, it's packed full of benefits such as vitamins C and E, as well as being a powerful anti-inflammatory and digestive aid. And, as many women know, cranberries are a powerful supplement that help with urinary tract infections.

To sweeten this combo up, I add a healthy dose of another North American favorite, Vermont maple syrup, plus a splash of fresh-pressed apple cider, making for a sweet, tart elixir that's sure to put the pep back in your step.

2 milliliters (40 drops) American ginseng extract

1 ounce (30 ml) unsweetened real cranberry juice

1 ounce (30 ml) fresh-pressed apple cider or juice

½ ounce (15 ml) Grade-A Vermont maple syrup

YIELD: 1 SHOT

Add all the ingredients to your cocktail shaker or mason jar. Shake hard to combine. Strain into a glass of your choice and enjoy.

NOTES

I don't use ice in this recipe because it dilutes the mix too much, but feel free to add 1 or 2 ice cubes if you prefer a less tangy flavor.

I often have a supply of this recipe mixed up in the fridge so I can just grab and go. As long as it's chilled, it should last up to 5 days.

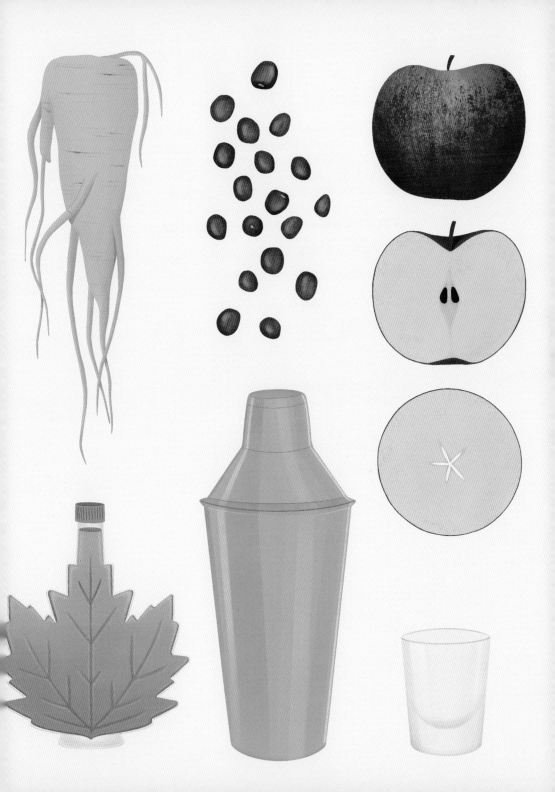

No-Bull Energy Shot

A rather famous energy drink company reached out to me years ago to ask if I'd be interested in helping them remake their formula. Their goal was to invent something more craft mixology-friendly and therefore appeal to the growing audience of "bar nerds." Of course, the thing about craft cocktail makers and bar nerds is that they demand fresh and mostly natural ingredients, conceived via time-honored, small-batch traditions. Needless to say, the makers of this mass-produced, artificial ingredient-based drink were not interested in hearing that they would need to consider using a much less chemically based recipe.

But by then the idea for this had started to percolate, so I decided to carry on with my R&D. To keep the base color as close as possible to the original, I chose an infusion of jasmine green tea. To this I added a powerhouse trio of adaptogens—ashwagandha, known for its restorative properties, rhodiola for its ability to increase mental clarity, enhance memory, and knock out anxiety and depression, and maca as a mood enhancer and immune booster.

To finish it off, I added a shot of vitamin B_{12}, one of my favorite supplements to help get me through a long day, and ginger-honey syrup. Because the plan was to carbonate this shot, I also added malic acid. The final result of all these efforts was a shot that provides the "wings" you're looking for—minus the harsh chemicals.

This recipe takes some time to come together, but it doesn't include anything that is hyper-perishable. It's the perfect weekend warrior project—make a batch and have it ready in the fridge for the week ahead.

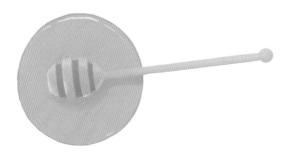

FOR THE HONEY GINGER SYRUP

1 cup (8 oz or 235 ml) runny honey

1 cup (8 oz or 235 ml) boiling water

¾ cup (180 g) peeled, chopped fresh ginger root

FOR THE NO-BULL ENERGY SHOT

3 bags jasmine green tea

1½ cups (12 oz or 355 ml) boiling water

½ ounce (1 tablespoon plus 20 drops or 15 ml) ashwagandha extract

1 teaspoon plus 12 drops (112 drops or 5.6 ml) rhodiola extract

¼ ounce (160 drops or 8 ml) maca extract

¼ ounce (160 drops or 8 ml) liquid vitamin B_{12}

5 ounces (150 ml) Honey Ginger Syrup

Scant ½ ounce (15 ml) apple cider vinegar

1 ounce (30 ml) malic acid solution (see Notes)

TO MAKE THE HONEY GINGER SYRUP: Add all the ingredients to a high-speed blender and blitz for about 30 seconds. Strain before using and store in the fridge until ready to use. This will keep in the fridge for up to 2 weeks.

TO MAKE THE NO-BULL ENERGY SHOT: Steep the tea bags in hot water in a teapot for 1 hour. Allow to cool completely before transferring to the fridge to chill. (Do not use ice to speed up the cooling process—you will have way too much dilution of flavor.)

Remove the tea bags and add the chilled tea and remaining ingredients to an airtight container and chill again for about 8 hours. You can place this in your freezer for the last hour before carbonating to help create more bubbles—just be careful it doesn't turn into a solid block.

TO SERVE: Pour the drink into your carbonator. Charge with CO_2 and allow the bubbles to subside. Open carefully so you don't lose half of your drink—it's like a shaken bottle of soda, so go slowly. Pour into a 2-ounce (60-ml) shot glass and enjoy!

NOTES

Regarding B_{12}: This stuff is incredibly potent, so use it sparingly and not too late in the day unless you're planning on staying up into the wee hours. I've made that mistake and found myself cleaning my oven at 3 a.m. like a maniac.

To make the malic acid solution, stir ½ teaspoon malic acid into 1 ounce (30 ml) of hot water.

"In Like a Lion" Serotonin Shot

For our final autumnal afternoon glow shot, I thought I'd bring you something a little fun. The glow shots in this book are shots, after all, so why not do one modeled after the classic car bomb–style beer-and-a shot combination—using nonalcoholic beer, of course.

The serotonin-boosting adaptogenic star of this show is lion's mane, a powerful mushroom that reduces anxiety and depression to a relic of the past while promoting brain function and concentration. I add this to a fruity, tart, spicy tonic of Alphonso mango puree, fresh lime juice, and chile or cayenne pepper. Drink the shot on its own or add it to a nonalcoholic pilsner of your choice. Either way, I'm sure you'll enjoy this new way to "do shots!"

Lime wedge and cayenne pepper or Tajín, for the rim

1.5 milliliters (30 drops) lion's mane extract

1 ounce (30 ml) Alphonso mango puree

½ ounce (15 ml) fresh-squeezed lime juice

½ ounce (15 ml) chilled simple syrup (see Note)

Pinch of sea salt

1 bottle of your favorite nonalcoholic pilsner (optional)

YIELD: 1 SHOT

Rim a shot glass with the lime wedge, invert the glass, and dip the rim in the pepper mix. Set it aside.

Add all the liquid ingredients, except the nonalcoholic beer and pinch of salt, to your cocktail shaker or mason jar with a lid. Shake for 5 seconds. Pour into a rimmed glass.

Either shoot the shot or drop it into a glass of nonalcoholic beer and drink up!

NOTE

Make the simple syrup for this recipe ahead of time. Mix equal parts cane sugar and hot water, stirring until the sugar dissolves completely. Allow to cool before using, and refrigerate it to store.

Albizia Holy Basil "Shambrusco"

My all-time favorite bubbly wine is the Italian sparkling red known as lambrusco. Made in the Emilia-Romagna region, it ranges from dry to fruity sweet and features dark red fruit flavors of cherries and blackberries, with a hint of violet. Since I stopped drinking, I've been tinkering with a few booze-free recipes, hoping to recreate this delightful effervescent refreshment. I think I've hit on a winner with this one, which uses a combination of tart pomegranate-cherry juice with a subtle floral finish.

Albizia and holy basil are my adaptogens here, with albizia serving as a nerve tonic helping to combat stress as well as aid with sleep, and holy basil functioning as an all-around mood and immune booster.

Because this is a carbonated drink, I recommend giving the formula at least eight hours of chilling time before hitting it with CO_2. As with the No-Bull recipe earlier in this chapter, you can also place the drink in the freezer for that last hour before it gets spritzed. That way you're increasing the likelihood of the fizz staying longer and creating more bubbles. Make a batch and keep it on hand for when you need a crushable nightcap, or serve at your next pizza party and thrill all your friends.

4 milliliters (80 drops) albizia extract

4 milliliters (80 drops) holy basil extract

1¾ cups plus 2 tablespoons (15 oz or 450 ml) unsweetened pomegranate-cherry juice (see Note)

5 ounces (150 ml) chamomile tea

2 to 4 ounces (60 to 120 ml) chilled simple syrup (to taste, see Note, page 34)

6 ounces (175 ml) red verjus

1 ounce (30 ml) rose water, such as Al Wadi brand

1 ounce (30 ml) malic acid solution (see Note, page 109)

YIELD: 4 TO 5 DRINKS

Add all the ingredients to a pitcher and stir. If desired, pour the drink into a bottle with a screw-top lid or just leave it in the pitcher. Chill in the fridge for at least 8 hours, or chill in the fridge for 7 hours and transfer to the freezer for the last hour.

Pour a serving of the drink into your carbonator and add bubbles. Pour into a glass and drink immediately, as the fizz will start to dissipate as the bubbles escape.

NOTE

If you can't find pomegranate-cherry juice, then combine 1 cup plus 3 tablespoons plus 3 teaspoons (10 oz or 285 ml) of pomegranate juice and 5 ounces (150 ml) of tart cherry juice as a substitute.

Moringa Unicorn Latte

This vibrant tea latte gets its amazing color from a botanical called butterfly blue pea flower, which you can find either as a whole dried flower or as a powder. The powder can be whipped into warm milk with a handy dandy milk frother. Butterfly blue pea flower has a subtle flavor by itself, so I steep some chamomile lavender tea or even just some food-grade lavender buds in hot water for extra flavor and peaceful vibes. And of course, I like to take things to the next level and add anxiety-fighting supplements, as well as dragon fruit powder and pastry glitter, for a complete body, mind, and eye-candy experience.

Moringa is the leading lady adaptogen in this fairytale-colored latte, bringing tranquility to your taste buds with every sip. Depending on how in need of sleep you are, you could also add rhodiola and ashwagandha, as I do sometimes. But moringa on its own tends to do the trick in this milky latte, helping you wind down and returning your brain to a baseline level of pure chill.

FOR THE MORINGA UNICORN LATTE

1 chamomile lavender tea bag or 1 teaspoon food-grade lavender flowers

2 ounces (60 ml) hot water

½ teaspoon butterfly blue pea tea powder, plus more for serving

5 ounces (150 ml) plant milk of your choice

½ ounce (15 ml) runny honey

1 drop real vanilla extract

1 milliliter (20 drops) moringa extract

FOR SERVING

Dragon fruit powder

Silver pastry glitter

Freshly grated nutmeg (optional)

YIELD: 1 LATTE

TO MAKE THE MORINGA UNICORN LATTE: In an 8-ounce (235-ml) cup, add the chamomile lavender tea bag and 2 ounces (60 ml) of boiling hot water. Steep the tea for 5 minutes; this also serves to warm up your latte cup!

Once steeped, remove the tea bag or lavender flowers and pour the hot tea into a small saucepan. Add the butterfly blue pea tea powder to the water and stir to make a slurry. Add the plant milk and honey and set it over low heat, stirring until the blue powder dissolves. Add the vanilla and moringa and use a milk frother to fully combine.

TO SERVE: Pour your latte into your heated cup. Sprinkle with butterfly blue pea powder and dragon fruit powder and swirl the surface with a toothpick. Dust with silver pastry glitter and grated nutmeg (if using).

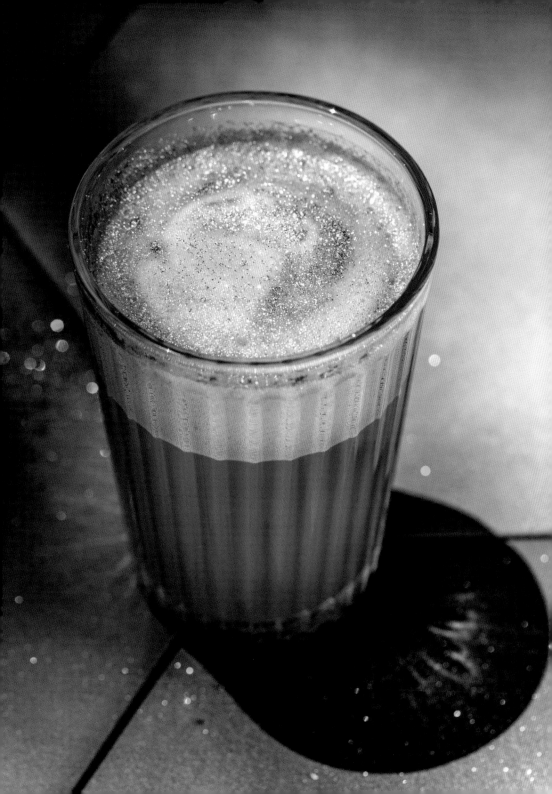

Reishi & Maca "Sleepy Time" Cosmo

Back in the 90s I lived in the New York City neighborhood where Sex and the City was filmed. Every week, my girlfriends and I gathered to watch the latest episode while sipping on Carrie's favorite cocktail: the cosmopolitan.

Now, my friend group is spread out all over the world—and none of us drink anymore. But should we ever get together, I'll serve my nonalcoholic "Sleepy Time" Cosmo. Naturally, this drink includes cranberry juice and lime, but my twist comes from adding chai spices and apple cider—plus maca, for its mood-enhancing and immune-boosting properties, and reishi, for its ability to quell anxiety and bring about restful sleep.

FOR THE CHAI-SPICED APPLE CIDER

1 cup (8 oz or 235 ml) fresh-pressed apple cider

¼ teaspoon ground cinnamon

½ teaspoon ground ginger

¼ teaspoon ground green cardamom

¼ teaspoon freshly grated nutmeg

Pinch of ground cloves

Pinch of fresh black pepper

FOR THE REISHI & MACA "SLEEPY TIME" COSMO

0.7 milliliter (14 drops) reishi extract

1 milliliter (20 drops) maca extract

1 ounce (30 ml) unsweetened real cranberry juice

2 ounces (60 ml) Chai-spiced Apple Cider

¾ ounce (22 ml) fresh-squeezed lime juice

¾ ounce (22 ml) chilled simple syrup (see Note)

3 dashes nonalcoholic orange bitters

1 drop real vanilla extract

1 orange twist

FOR SERVING

Lime wheel (optional)

YIELD: 1 COSMO

TO MAKE THE CHAI-SPICED APPLE CIDER: Add all the ingredients to a heavy-bottomed pan over low heat and heat through for about 5 minutes. Allow to sit for 30 minutes, then strain through a fine-mesh strainer and chill before using.

TO MAKE THE "SLEEPY TIME" COSMO: Add all ingredients, including the orange twist, with 5 ice cubes to your cocktail shaker or mason jar with a lid. Shake for 10 seconds.

TO SERVE: Strain into a chilled martini or coupe glass and garnish with a lime wheel.

NOTE

Make the simple syrup for this recipe ahead of time. Mix equal parts cane sugar and hot water, stirring until the sugar dissolves completely. Allow to cool before using, and refrigerate.

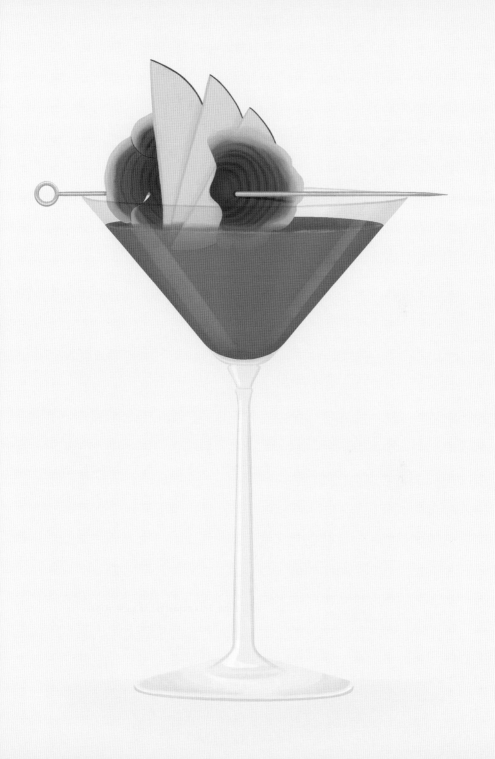

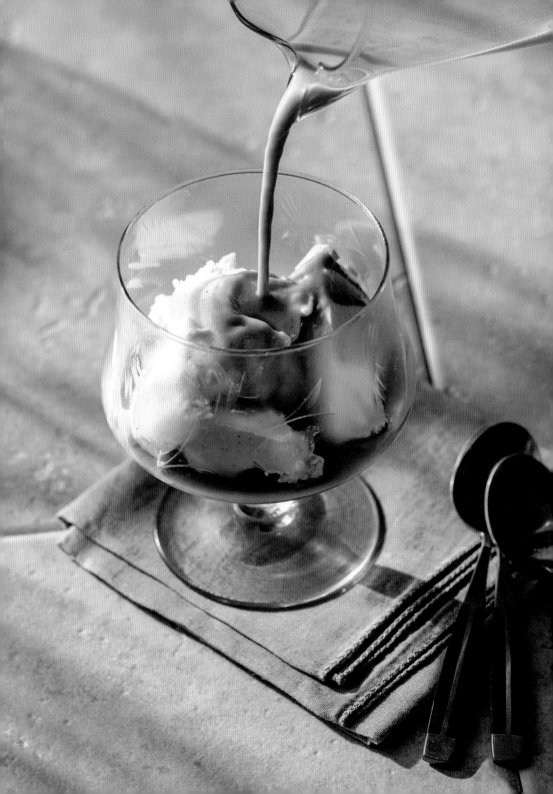

Matcha Affogato

This next adaptogenic treat might seem like an odd choice for the cooler months, but with its warming gingery spices and soothing green tea flavors, I think you'll find it's actually the perfect end to a meal any time of the year. The inspiration for this affogato comes from two sources: a traditional affogato, which is topped with espresso, and a tropical piña colada.

Bear with me, and I will have you drooling to try this. An affogato is generally made with vanilla ice cream or gelato. For this recipe, I use homemade coconut pineapple ice cream instead, which is beyond divine, if I may say so. If you don't want to go to the trouble of making your own ice cream, you can use a store-bought version. Plain store-bought coconut ice cream will also do in a pinch.

Instead of coffee, we use matcha green tea to "drown" our ice cream. The grassiness of the green tea and the fruitiness of the pineapple pair beautifully together. And for added complexity, I add a healthy dose of ground ginger and nutmeg.

As for the adaptogens in this blissful blend, I've chosen astragalus and ashwagandha for their combined ability to bring calm to the mind and help with immunity, recovery, and peaceful sleep. After this affogato, you can't help but have beautiful dreams!

FOR THE COCONUT PINEAPPLE ICE CREAM

3 cups (465 g) fresh pineapple cubes

1 can (13.5 ounces or 398 ml) full-fat coconut milk

⅔ cup (132 g) cane sugar

1 ounce (30 ml) fresh-squeezed lime juice

½ teaspoon real vanilla extract

½ teaspoon coconut extract (optional)

continued on next page

YIELD: 1 SERVING

TO MAKE THE COCONUT PINEAPPLE ICE CREAM: Add all the ingredients to your blender and combine until smooth. Pour mixture into a loaf pan and chill for about 4 hours. Scrape mixture back into the blender and pulse. Transfer the mix into an ice cream maker and freeze according to your machine's instructions. Store in the freezer with a layer of parchment paper over the top to prevent ice crystals from forming on the surface.

continued on next page

FOR THE MATCHA AFFOGATO

2 teaspoons matcha
green tea powder

½ teaspoon ground ginger

3 ounces (90 ml) hot water

2 milliliters (40 drops)
ashwagandha extract

2 milliliters (40 drops)
astragalus root extract

FOR SERVING

2 scoops Coconut
Pineapple Ice Cream

Freshly grated nutmeg

TO MAKE THE MATCHA AFFOGATO: In a small bowl, use a fork to whisk together the matcha green tea and ginger. Add a teaspoon of water and mix it into a paste. Slowly add the remaining hot water, and use a milk frother now to whisk as you go, until all the lumps have dissolved and the matcha is nice and smooth. Add the ashwagandha and astragalus to the matcha and stir to combine.

TO SERVE: Pour the warm spiced matcha over the ice cream, and grate some fresh nutmeg on top.

NOTE

An affogato starts out as a dessert, but as the ice cream and matcha melt together it turns into a luscious drink. Keep that spoon handy so you can scrape up any leftovers at the bottom of the glass!

Superberry Punch

As the year starts to wind down, all manner of festivities begin popping up on your calendar. For folks like me—and I assume you too—there aren't many nonalcoholic beverage options on the celebration table. Us nondrinkers tend to get left out of the fun with minimal options beyond bubble water.

So instead of showing up to your next Thanksgiving bash with a four pack of ginger ale, how about trying this delightful goji berry–laced punch to brighten up your and everyone else's night? Adaptogenic goji berries as I've mentioned before, are a powerful antioxidant rich in phytonutrients, vitamins A and C, and minerals. Hence why many experts call them superberries. In fact, goji berries are widely revered in Traditional Chinese Medicine, so much so that Himalayan monks it is rumored, steep them in hot water to help give them stamina during long sessions of mediation.

To up the berry ante, I also include schisandra berry in this recipe, to help support anxiety-ridden wallflowers, as well as boost immunity ahead of cold season. The berry fest is completed by healthful, tart, bright cranberries and complemented by fresh apple cider, fragrant orange oil, and cinnamon sticks. This radiant celebratory punch will for sure be the life of any party worth going to!

6 ounces (175 ml) Goji
Berry Juice (page 55)

2 teaspoons plus 40 drops
(240 drops or 12 ml)
schisandra berry extract

1½ cups (12 oz or 355 ml)
unsweetened real cranberry juice

2¼ cups (18 oz or 540 ml) fresh-pressed apple cider

6 ounces (175 ml) Grade-A
Vermont maple syrup

6 to 8 whole cinnamon sticks

6 to 8 slices navel orange,
plus more for garnish

6 drops real vanilla extract

FOR SERVING

Orange slices, for garnish
(optional)

YIELD: 6 TO 8 SERVINGS

Combine all the ingredients in a large, airtight container or pitcher. Transfer to the fridge and allow to steep for up to 8 hours so all the oils from the cinnamon and oranges infuse the punch.

TO SERVE: Transfer to a punch bowl and ladle into punch cups. Garnish with a slice of orange, if desired.

Rosy Glow Horchata with Shiitake & Velvet Bean

This version of the Mexican favorite horchata is a delish way to bring a glow to your next party or gathering, thanks to the adaptogenic shiitake mushrooms and velvet bean. In Traditional Chinese Medicine, shiitakes are known for bringing virility, youthfulness, and energy to the body while also being a powerful immune booster. As for velvet bean, it's an excellent supplement to take for increasing dopamine and fighting anxiety.

Given that shiitakes are widely used in Traditional Chinese Medicine, I thought I would stick to a theme and use Chinese five-spice powder as a substitute for cinnamon in the horchata. This culinary blend does include cinnamon, but also star anise, cloves, fennel seeds, and Szechuan peppercorn. We finish with a hint of rose water on the palate to make for a vibrant and refreshing pitcher of goodness!

2 teaspoons plus 40 drops (240 drops or 12 ml) shiitake extract

¾ teaspoon velvet bean powder

1 teaspoon Chinese five-spice powder

6 cups (48 oz or 1.44 L) unsweetened rice milk

6 ounces (175 ml) chilled simple syrup (see Note)

1½ ounces (45 ml) rose water, such as Al Wadi brand

¼ teaspoon sea salt

Freshly grated nutmeg, for serving

YIELD: 6 TO 8 SERVINGS

Add all the ingredients to your blender and blend on high for 30 seconds. Adjust the sweetness level to taste and pour into a pitcher. Serve over ice with grated nutmeg on the top.

NOTE
Make the simple syrup for this recipe ahead of time. Mix equal parts cane sugar and hot water, stirring until the sugar dissolves completely. Allow to cool before using, and refrigerate it to store.

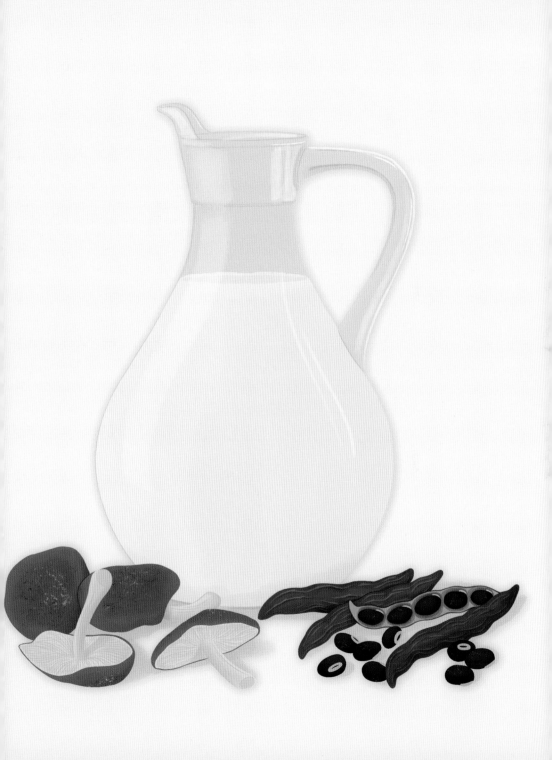

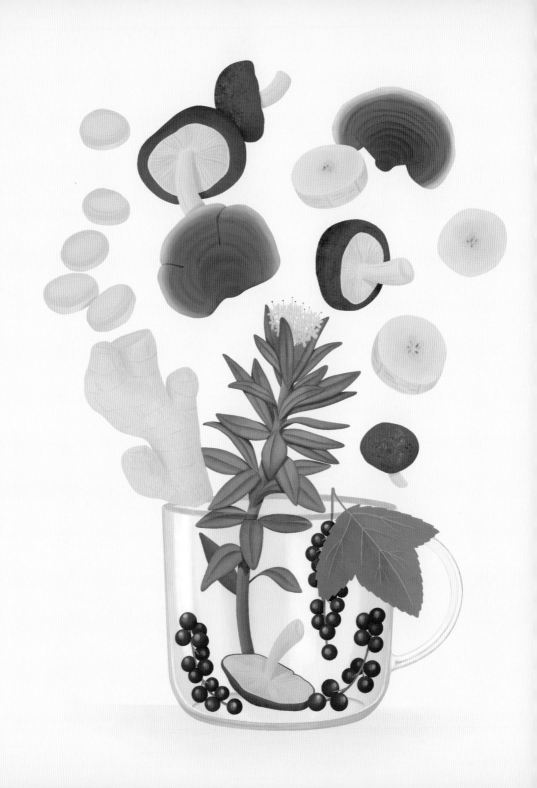

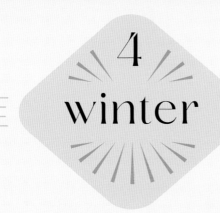

4
winter

Winter officially begins on December 21st, but if you live in the United States, it really starts the last Thursday in November when Thanksgiving kicks off the start of the holiday season. A parade of festivities follows over the next five weeks. It's a time when people gather together after a long year, families reuniting from all over the world, bringing a sense of joy . . . and stress at the same time.

There can be a lot of anxiety at this time of year, and depression as well, thanks to long hours of travel, overspending, or family conflicts. It doesn't help that winter means shorter days and a dearth of sunshine (a wonder drug, in my opinion) and its vitamin D goodness. As well as getting vitamin fixes, I find that increasing the use of adaptogenic supplements such as turmeric, reishi, chaga, and velvet bean becomes critical to surviving the holidays and beyond.

The adaptogen-infused recipes in this chapter are similar to the comfort-focused brews from autumn, but they feature adaptogenic blends designed to put a different kind of glow in your cheeks. In this chapter, you'll see a lot more blends with ashitaba, amla, and pine pollen to target depression and boost focus, energy, and immunity. Or bacopa and shiitake, which battle stress and anxiety, as well as increase virility and youthfulness.

I've reinvented a few holiday classics here, including my own plant-based version of Irish cream (yep, that's right, I reinvented Baileys for the dairy-free crowd). I also reinvented the (unfortunately named) Porn Star Martini, billed as the world's favorite cocktail and, in my opinion, the perfect way to ring in the New Year without the hard stuff.

It's my hope that with these adaptogenic drinks, winter will be the time of joy and rest that it's supposed to be, instead of a season of stress and sadness. I wish that all your holidays are infused with bright moods and much light. Cheers!

Big Boost
Banana Smoothie

One of my favorite ways to start the day is with bananas and maple syrup. Usually, this takes the form of a banana pancake, essentially ripe bananas mashed up with a raw egg and shredded coconut and fried like a traditional silver dollar pancake. Dipped in maple syrup, "banana cakes" are just divine and an excellent way to get your morning protein fix.

But what if I don't have time to cook up this delightful breakfast dish?

Enter the Big Boost Banana Smoothie, which uses healthy doses of adaptogens ashitaba, amla, and pine pollen. Ashitaba, known in Japan as the longevity herb, is packed with vitamins B_6 and B_{12}, enough to energize any sleepy bunny and help with digestion. Amla contributes its ability to fight the blues and enhance performance, while pine pollen improves cognitive function and supports immunity.

As it's winter, I recommend using fresh rather than frozen bananas here, so your smoothie stays at a comfortable room temperature. And make sure not to skip the maple syrup and nutmeg! That extra dose of flavor turns this healthful drink into a craveable one.

1 teaspoon ashitaba powder

1 teaspoon amla powder

1 teaspoon pine pollen powder

1 ripe banana

¼ cup (38 g) ripe
fresh blueberries

1 teaspoon unsweetened
shredded coconut

1 teaspoon unrefined coconut oil

6 ounces (175 ml) full-fat coconut
milk or milk of your choice

1 ounce (30 ml) Grade-A
Vermont maple syrup

¼ teaspoon freshly
grated nutmeg

YIELD: 1 SMOOTHIE

Add all the ingredients to your blender and blitz on high for about 30 seconds. Transfer to a cup or glass of your choice and reap the rewards of a nourishing breakfast!

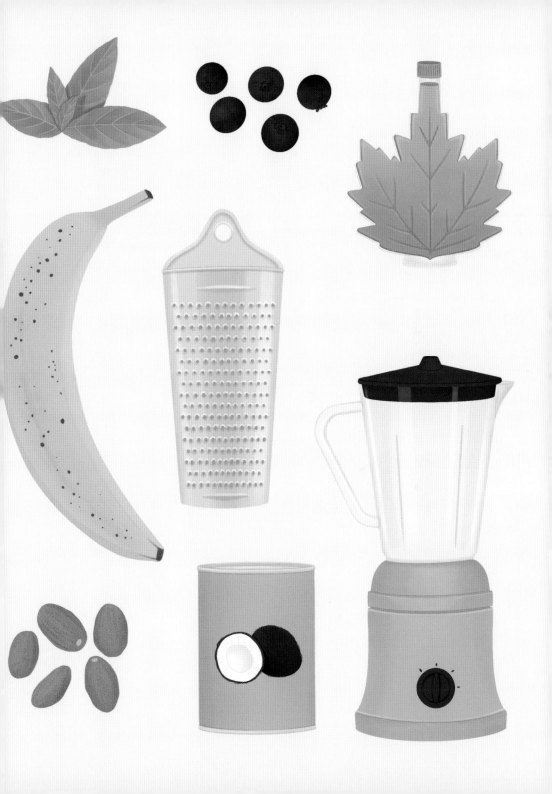

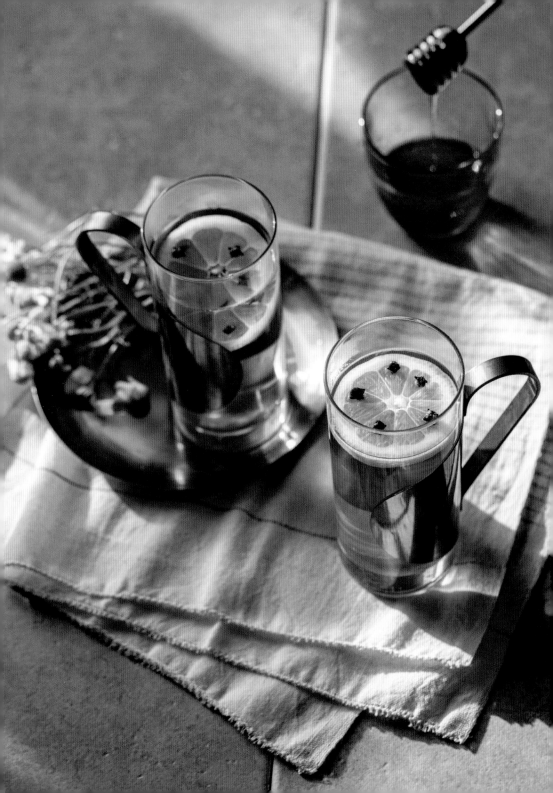

Morning, Sunshine! Gotu Kola Toddy

I used to love warming up in the winter with a hot toddy. But since I gave up alcohol, I've been making a booze-free version based on the toddies my pops would make for me as a kiddo when I was fighting a cold. My pops was a master of the toddy, often mixing up odd concoctions of warmed up Guinness beer, honey, and spices for himself. The PG-version he served me was mostly a squeeze of fresh lemon juice, with the husk it was squeezed from, tossed in a mug with a generous spoon full of thick Linden blossom honey, a weak infusion of hot tea, and an orange peel studded with dried cloves. On occasion, a pinch of cayenne pepper made its way in there too to induce "the sweats" to purge infection.

In my updated version of this childhood favorite, I use Japanese yuzu juice. Yuzu is a citrus that's a cross between a lemon and a mandarin orange; its juice has a beautiful, bright floral quality to it. For the adaptogenic additions, I chose gotu kola to help with cognitive health, stress, and anxiety, and shatavari for its vibrational and immune-boosting abilities.

1 milliliter (20 drops) gotu kola extract

0.7 milliliter (14 drops) shatavari extract

1 cup (8 oz or 235 ml) hot chamomile, jasmine green, or oolong tea

¾ ounce (22 ml) yuzu citrus juice or fresh-squeezed lemon juice

1 ounce (30 ml) runny honey

1 drop real vanilla extract

Orange peel, for garnish

YIELD: 1 TODDY

Add all the ingredients to a mug and stir until the honey dissolves. Garnish with an orange peel and enjoy.

"Do the Mochamotion" Mushroom Latte

As a young barista behind the counter of one of the more popular coffee shops in New York City, my most dreaded order was a mocha latte. The sticky chocolate syrup that refused to completely dissolve in my milk frothing pitcher made such a mess.

These days when I mix up a café mocha, I prefer to use a rich dark chocolate with maximum cocoa solids and minimal sugar. The rich flavors of good-quality chocolate pair divinely with the earthy, fragrant tones of mushrooms—specifically, energy-promoting and anxiety-kicking reishi, which helps with focus and cognitive function, or shiitakes, with their ability to boost virility, immunity, and energy levels.

To create this recipe, use either the liquid extracts of each of these fungi individually or opt for a powdered mushroom blend that incorporates all of them.

FOR THE "DO THE MOCHAMOTION" MUSHROOM LATTE

1 cup (8 oz or 235 ml) oat or cashew milk, or milk of your choice

Pinch of sea salt

Pinch of cayenne pepper

1 ounce (30 ml) espresso

1 scoop (1000 mg) powdered mushroom blend OR 1 milliliter (20 drops) each of reishi, lion's mane, and shiitake extracts

1 ounce (30 ml) simple syrup (see Note)

1 ounce (28 g) good-quality dark chocolate or a teaspoon of cocoa powder

FOR SERVING

1 spoonful of crème fraiche (optional)

Pinch of ground cinnamon

YIELD: 1 MOCHA LATTE

TO MAKE THE "DO THE MOCHAMOTION" MUSHROOM LATTE: In a small heavy-bottomed saucepan, add the milk, pinch of sea salt, cayenne, and espresso. Place over low heat to warm through, about 3 minutes or so. Don't let it come to a boil; it will burn.

Once warmed, add the mushroom blend, simple syrup, and chocolate, and use a milk frother to blend slowly until the chocolate dissolves.

TO SERVE: Pour latte into a warmed mug and add a dollop of crème fraiche and a pinch of cinnamon.

NOTE

Make the simple syrup for this recipe ahead of time. Mix equal parts cane sugar and hot water, stirring until the sugar dissolves completely. Allow to cool before using, and refrigerate it to store.

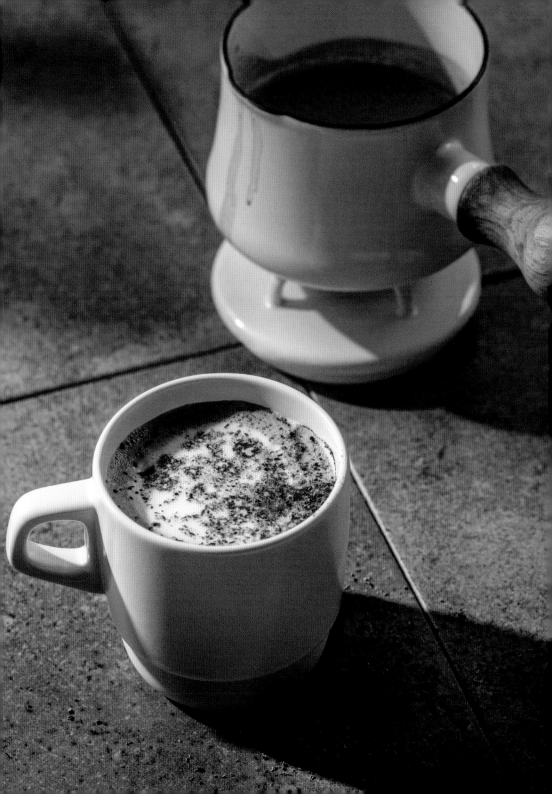

Rising Sun Shake

This next recipe takes its cues from golden milk, a popular drink you can find in many juice bars. Taking center stage here is turmeric, with its depression-fighting and mood-boosting superpowers. You can find turmeric root, as well as fresh ginger, in most good supermarkets and Southeast Asian stores. If you can't find fresh turmeric root, the ground version works just as well to create that inner glow; however, the flavor will be much more muted.

This delicious, warming drink features a potent blend of dynamic adaptogens: ginger aids with digestion, cordyceps promotes energy as well as immune support, and, of course, the golden root itself. It is the perfect fix for those wintery morning blues. Even if the sun isn't shining on you from above, it will definitely shine on you from within!

FOR THE TURMERIC-GINGER SYRUP

¼ cup (60 g) fresh peeled turmeric root or 2 tablespoons (30 g) ground turmeric

½ cup (120 g) peeled, chopped fresh ginger root

2 cups (16 oz or 475 ml) honey

2 cups (16 oz or 475 ml) hot water

FOR THE RISING SUN SHAKE

1 ounce (30 ml) Turmeric-Ginger Syrup

1½ milliliters (30 drops) cordyceps extract

1 cup (8 oz or 235 ml) cashew milk or plant-based milk of your choice

Pinch of ground allspice

Pinch of sea salt

Orange peel, for oil spritzing

YIELD: 1 SHAKE

TO MAKE THE TURMERIC-GINGER SYRUP: Add all the ingredients to your blender and blend on high for about 30 seconds. Strain though a fine-mesh strainer, pushing the liquid through the solids with the back of a tablespoon or small ladle. Store in an airtight container in the fridge for up to 7 days.

TO MAKE THE RISING SUN SHAKE: Add all the ingredients, except the orange peel, to your blender. Pulse 4 to 5 times to incorporate, then pour into a glass of your choice. Alternatively, add everything directly to the glass and whip it up with a milk frother. Spritz a little oil from an orange peel over the top of the shake for an extra kick of sunshine.

NOTE
Don't save this recipe just for winter. During summer or in warmer climates, substitute three scoops of plant-based ice cream for the plant milk and blend together for a proper thick milkshake.

Kola & Tonic

Back in the mid-aughts, a Swedish barista invented a new way of getting your afternoon caffeine fix. He mixed espresso with tonic water, thus giving birth to a brew that you can now find all over Europe and South America; less so in the United States. It might sound like an odd choice, but the citrus notes in the tonic water perfectly complement the aromatics in the coffee and balance some of the bitterness. It's an excellent midday pick-me-up any time of the year, but my version, which incorporates green cardamom bitters, is especially enjoyable in the winter.

I include a recipe here for nonalcoholic cardamom bitters, but it's more of a weekend project than a "hey, presto!" situation, as you'll have to hunt down some ingredients. Because cardamom bitters make everything better (a simple glass of carrot juice with cardamom bitters is absolutely divine), I don't mind using a store-bought brand with a small amount of alcohol if I don't have time to make my own.

For the adaptogens here I chose Siberian ginseng and gotu kola. The ginseng dials up your mental alertness to a ten and improves endurance, while gotu kola dials down your stress and anxiety levels to almost nothing.

The bonus here is that you need no fancy tools to get your Kola & Tonic on: Just pop open a bottle, pour, and be refreshed!

**FOR THE NONALCOHOLIC
CARDAMOM BITTERS**

2 ounces (60 ml) burnt sugar or caramel syrup

5 ounces (150 ml) warm water

4 drops cardamom oil

4 drops Fiori di Sicilia oil

½ ounce (15 ml) alcohol-free gentian extract

FOR THE KOLA & TONIC

1 ounce (30 ml) cold brew concentrate
or chilled espresso

1 milliliter (20 drops) Siberian ginseng extract

1 milliliter (20 drops) gotu kola extract

3 dashes homemade nonalcoholic cardamom
bitters or regular store-bought bitters

6 ounces (175 ml) tonic water

Orange twist, for garnish

--- **YIELD: 1 APERITIF** ---

**TO MAKE THE NONALCOHOLIC
CARDAMOM BITTERS:** Add all the ingredients to a glass or mason jar. Either blend with a small milk frother or shake hard to combine. Store in an airtight bottle in the fridge for up to 3 months.

TO MAKE THE KOLA & TONIC: Add the cold brew, ginseng, gotu kola, and bitters to a highball or other tall glass. Add ice and top with tonic water. Garnish with an orange twist.

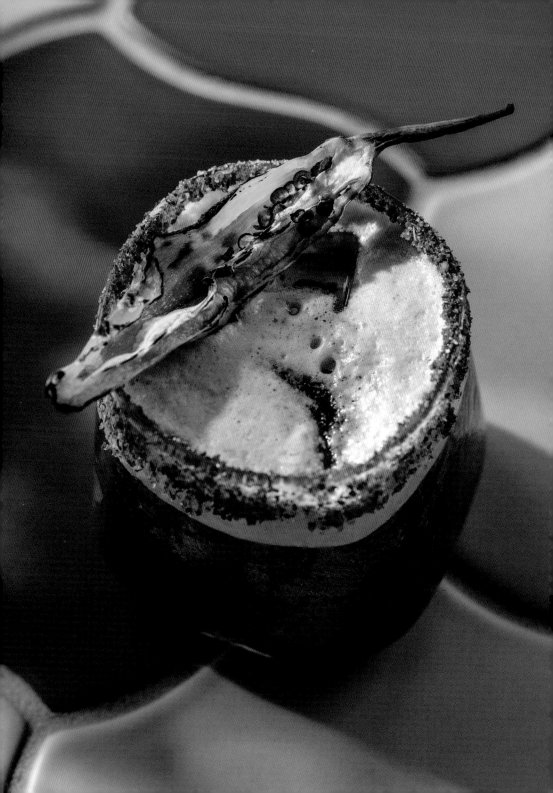

Sangresandra "Margarita"

In my years as a drink slinger, the two most popular cocktails that I made were both margaritas, one of which featured a combo of blood orange and jalapeño. My nonalcoholic sangresandra "margarita" takes its cues from this drink. In Spanish, *sangre* means blood, while *sandra* I've taken from that adaptogenic marvel, schisandra berry. Unlike some adaptogens, schisandra berry assists the body on several fronts. First, as an anxiety tamer, helping to lighten the load; second, as a powerful immune supporter; and last, but not least, as an energizer, boosting endurance to get you through the longest of days.

I pair it in this recipe with my MVP, holy basil, for its ability to turn that frown upside down almost immediately, making sure that you can get through the rest of your day with grace and ease!

FOR THE SANGRESANDRA "MARGARITA"

1 to 2 slices jalapeño pepper, seeds removed

Pinch of sea salt

1 ounce (30 ml) simple syrup (see Note)

2 milliliters (40 drops) schisandra berry extract

0.7 milliliters (14 drops) holy basil extract

1½ ounces (45 ml) fresh-squeezed blood orange juice

½ ounce (15 ml) fresh-squeezed lime juice

1 ounce (30 ml) unsweetened pineapple juice or filtered water

FOR SERVING

Sea salt or Tajín, for the rim (optional)

Charred pepper, for garnish (optional)

YIELD: 1 "MARGARITA"

TO MAKE THE SANGRESANDRA "MARGARITA": Add the jalapeño slices, salt, and simple syrup to your cocktail shaker or mason jar, and muddle with either the end of a wooden spoon or a muddler. Add the remaining ingredients and 5 ice cubes. Shake hard for 5 seconds.

TO SERVE: Strain into a chilled rocks glass that has been dusted on the rim with sea salt or Tajín. Add ice and garnish with a charred pepper if you're feeling extra fancy!

NOTE

Make the simple syrup for this recipe ahead of time. Mix equal parts cane sugar and hot water, stirring until the sugar dissolves completely. Allow to cool before using, and refrigerate it to store.

Turmeric Buck

The next recipe I present to you is a warming version of the popular Moscow mule, except, of course, without the vodka. Instead, the hit of heat comes from mood-lifting turmeric, with its earthy spiced tones, and its close cousin, ginger root. While ginger root is not classified as an adaptogen, it has a reputation for increasing both serotonin and dopamine almost as well as its golden-hued relative. The recipe also includes another adaptogenic marvel, chaga, with its ability to quell anxiety and promote both immunity and energy levels.

As for the name, mules are members of the Buck cocktail family. A Prohibition-era favorite, Bucks were known for serving up a kick on the back end from their gingery heat—much like a bucking mule. Enjoy this glowing elixir warmed through as a wintery toddy or chilled over ice any time for a mood-lifting fix!

FOR THE GINGER SYRUP

1 cup (240 g) peeled, chopped fresh ginger root

2 cups (400 g) cane sugar

2 cups (16 oz or 475 ml) hot water

FOR THE TURMERIC BUCK

1 milliliter (20 drops) chaga extract

0.7 milliliter (14 drops) turmeric extract

1 ounce (30 ml) fresh Ginger Syrup

1 ounce (30 ml) fresh-squeezed lemon juice

3 ounces (90 ml) fresh-pressed apple cider

½ teaspoon unsalted butter (optional)

Lemon slice, for serving

YIELD: 1 BUCK

TO MAKE THE GINGER SYRUP: Add all the ingredients to your blender and blend on high for about 30 seconds. Strain though a fine-mesh strainer, pushing the liquid through the solids with the back of a tablespoon or small ladle. Store in an airtight container in the fridge for up to 7 days.

TO MAKE THE TURMERIC BUCK: Add all the ingredients, except the lemon slice, to a heavy-bottomed pan. Place the pan over low heat and warm through, but do not allow to boil—about 3 minutes. Pour into a heatproof cup and garnish with a slice of lemon.

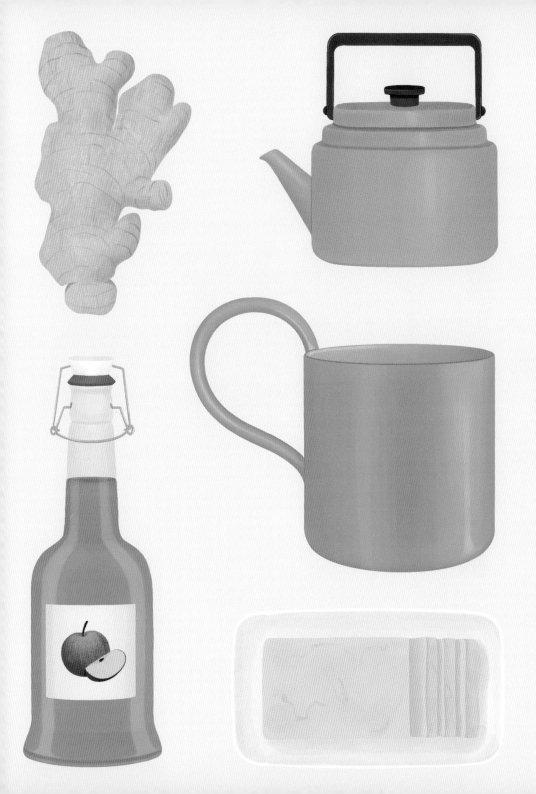

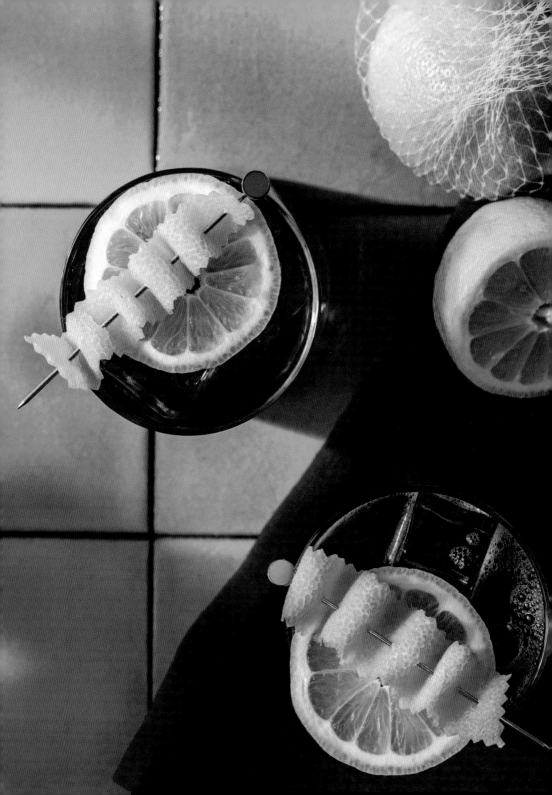

You Maca Me Crazy! Sour

This wintery riff on the classic summer refreshment, fresh lemonade, is just what the adaptogenic doc ordered, with its blend of mood-enhancing, immune-boosting maca and anxiety-busting moringa.

To give it that wintery holiday feel, real cranberry juice and apple cider vinegar join this healing party, bringing along high levels of antioxidants, vitamins, and digestive support. The touch of apple cider vinegar also brings with it cholesterol fighting superpowers, so it's the perfect postprandial digestif for any time of day. Add Vermont maple syrup imbued with cinnamon and allspice for that quintessential 'tis the season festive feel.

**FOR THE SPICED VERMONT
MAPLE SYRUP**

1½ cups (12 oz or 355 ml) Grade-A
Vermont maple syrup

Peel of 1 navel orange, cut into strips

4 whole cinnamon sticks

10 allspice berries

2 bay leaves

FOR THE YOU MACA ME CRAZY! SOUR

0.5 milliliter (10 drops) maca extract

1 milliliter (20 drops) moringa extract

2 ounces (60 ml) unsweetened
real cranberry juice

2 ounces (60 ml) chilled hibiscus tea
or filtered water

1 ounce (30 ml) fresh-squeezed lemon juice

½ ounce (15 ml) apple cider vinegar

1 ounce (30 ml) Spiced Vermont Maple Syrup

Lemon slice, for garnish

YIELD: 1 SOUR

**TO MAKE THE SPICED VERMONT MAPLE
SYRUP:** Add all the ingredients to a 16-ounce (475-ml) mason jar with a lid. Allow the syrup to sit and infuse for at least 5 days before using. There is no need to strain the infusing ingredients off; the longer you leave them, the more intense the resulting flavor. Store up to 1 month in the fridge and use as desired.

TO MAKE THE YOU MACA ME CRAZY! SOUR:
Add all the ingredients, except the lemon slice, with 5 ice cubes to your cocktail shaker or mason jar with a lid. Shake hard for 5 seconds. Strain into a chilled glass of your choice and fill with ice. Garnish with a slice of lemon and serve.

Ashitaba Energy Booster

This next recipe is a very quick fix for that midafternoon slump, featuring a healthy dose of ashitaba, which is chock-full of vitamins B_6 and B_{12}. Ashitaba is a flowering plant that is a member of the carrot family. Its name literally translates to "tomorrow's leaf." Often used for maladies such as indigestion, it is native to the Pacific coast of Japan and is believed to contribute to the longevity and health of the local residents. Ashitaba is available online and in many health food stores as a tea powder similar to matcha green tea powder, except that ashitaba is caffeine-free, making it the perfect midday energy boost that won't leave you amped up into the evening.

I love to whip ashitaba up with hot water, cashew milk, and a teaspoon of honey or maple syrup. I'll also often add in velvet bean for a dopamine boost, as well as a spritz of lemon oil to bring me a reviving burst of citrus that wakes up my senses.

½ teaspoon ashitaba tea powder

½ teaspoon velvet bean powder

4 ounces (120 ml) boiling water

½ ounce (15 ml) Grade-A Vermont maple syrup or honey

1 ounce (30 ml) cashew milk

Lemon twist, for oil spritzing

YIELD: 1 SHOT

Add the ashitaba and velvet bean powders to a heatproof cup. Pour in the boiling water. Whisk with a small fork until the powder dissolves or use a milk frother to ensure maximum absorption of the powder into the water. Add the maple syrup or honey and the milk and stir.

Spritz the oil from the lemon twist over the cup by pinching it between your thumb and finger. Enjoy!

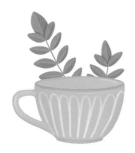

Sea Buck Immunity Shot

I'm a relative newcomer to the benefits of sea buckthorn, but so far I love, love, love what it does for my skin and joints. As someone who spends long hours on their feet, sea buckthorn oil has been a lifesaver, helping fight inflammation and soothe tired muscles. It also gives my winter skin a wonderous glow when used topically.

Known in Ayurveda and Traditional Chinese Medicine as the holy fruit of the Himalayas, this powerful adaptogen has been used for centuries for many ailments. Rich in essential compounds, such as vitamins A, C, and E, and the minerals zinc, calcium, and iron, sea buckthorn can be used for immune support too. I often add it to a veggie juice or smoothie, but if I'm on the go, I like to shoot it with coconut water, carrot, and orange juice, all of which are easy to find in most supermarkets.

I pair it here with camu camu, an Amazonian berry that's documented as containing the highest dose of vitamin C in the plant world. Because camu camu is a natural food source, it absorbs easier into the digestive system and won't irritate your tummy like some synthetic vitamin C brands can. You can find it at most health food stores, or, if you prefer to shop online, there are several outlets that stock it.

1 milliliter (20 drops) sea buckthorn oil

0.7 milliliter (14 drops) camu camu tincture

2 ounces (60 ml) carrot-orange juice (see Notes)

2 ounces (60 ml) virgin coconut water

YIELD: 1 SHOT

Add all the ingredients to a small glass and stir with a spoon. And shoot!

NOTES

Make the carrot-orange juice by juicing one carrot and half an orange together in your juicer. If you have a cold press juicer, juice extra and keep it for up to 2 days. If using a centrifugal spinning juicer, sadly, you will need to drink the juice immediately. You can also find this common juice blend in stores or online.

Bacopa Cup-a-Soup

As a kiddo, one of my favorite midwinter snacks when I got home from school was Cup-a-Soup. In case you're not familiar, this is a powdered soup to which you add boiling water. Nutritionally, it was pretty void of value. But it did feed my soul with its savory warmth and tide me over until dinnertime.

These days, when I need an instant soup fix, I turn to miso paste. Miso is popular in Japanese cuisine and is made from fermented soybeans and other ingredients such as koji, barley, seaweed, and salt. Add a heaping spoonful to boiling water in a pot, give it a few stirs, and voilà, your winter-worn self will be soothed.

Of course, I make a version with adaptogens to revive my body and restore my mind as well. I most often choose shiitake extract to boost my energy and immunity levels, but I also love bacopa, an Ayurvedic favorite. This flowering plant has been used for centuries to improve spatial learning and help focus the brain to support memory retention. It's also a valuable ally in taming stress and anxiety.

The great thing about miso, and this recipe in general, is that it's incredibly portable, meaning you can stash some miso in your office or school fridge and all you really need is a hot water kettle, a mug, and a spoon to put this rejuvenating delight together. At the same time, it can be gussied up with veggies, chicken, or tofu, and enhanced with, my fave, toasted sesame oil, for quite a satisfying light meal.

1 teaspoon organic white miso paste

4 ounces (120 ml) boiling water

2 milliliters (40 drops) shiitake extract

0.7 milliliters (14 drops) bacopa extract

1 thin slice fresh peeled ginger root (optional)

2 to 3 drops toasted sesame oil (optional)

YIELD: 1 DRINK

Add miso paste to a cup and add the boiling water. Stir to dissolve. You can also use a milk frother for faster mixing. Add shiitake and bacopa, as well as ginger root and sesame oil (if using), and stir to combine.

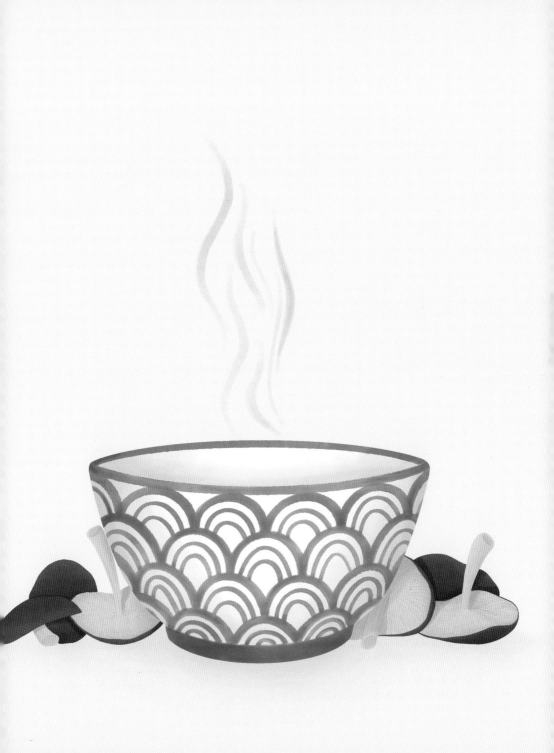

The MVP Shot

MVP, as most of us know, is the acronym for Most Valuable Player, but in this recipe it stands for Motivation, Vitality, and Pep (as in "in your step"). Rhodiola is covering the motivation and vitality here, with its ability to restore clarity, memory, and endurance, as well as kick anxiety, depression, and fatigue to the curb. As for the pep, that comes from the holy basil—its mood-enhancing properties have the ability to turn the deepest frown upside down!

0.7 milliliter (14 drops) rhodiola extract

0.7 milliliter (14 drops) holy basil extract

2 ounces (60 ml) unsweetened real pomegranate juice

½ ounce (15 ml) Grade-A Vermont maple syrup

Pinch of ground Saigon cinnamon

YIELD: 1 SHOT

Add all the ingredients to an 8-ounce (235-ml) mason jar. Shake with the lid on for about 10 seconds, until the maple syrup and cinnamon get fully incorporated into the juice. Remove the lid and drink immediately.

Reishi Ginger Nightcap

In the last couple of years, intermittent fasting has become a common, beneficial part of many people's health regimens. Personally, I try to make sure I have my last meal no later than 5 p.m., as I find it helps with digestion, as well as sleep. But sometimes, especially in the wintertime, that long fast between early dinner and next morning's breakfast can be a challenge. I find that a steaming hot mug of bone broth is the perfect answer to this problem, simultaneously soothing the mind for a great night's sleep and curbing hunger until morning without breaking the fast.

To make this more of a functional addition to my diet, I add a dose of reishi extract to help fight the winter blues, and albizia to reduce stress and improve sleep. Both also happen to be powerful immune boosters and antivirals, so they're perfect supplements to take if you are fighting a cold. I like to add toasted sesame oil and pho spices to my cup for added savory complexity, making this nightcap one of my favorite late-night winter rituals.

1 cup (8 oz or 235 ml) bone broth (see Notes)

1 slice fresh peeled ginger root

½ packet pho liquid concentrate (optional— see Notes)

Pinch of sea salt

1¼ milliliters (25 drops) reishi extract

0.7 milliliter (14 drops) albizia extract

2 to 3 drops toasted sesame oil

YIELD: 1 NIGHTCAP

Add the broth, ginger, pho concentrate, and sea salt to a small heavy-bottomed pan. Place the pan over low heat and bring to a simmer, allowing the ginger to steep for 5 minutes or so in the hot broth.

Remove from the heat and transfer to a heatproof mug. Add the reishi and albizia to the mug and stir. Finish by adding the toasted sesame oil.

NOTES

I make my own bone broth by boiling chicken bones, but you can easily substitute your favorite store-bought version.

You can find pho liquid concentrate in most good Asian markets or online.

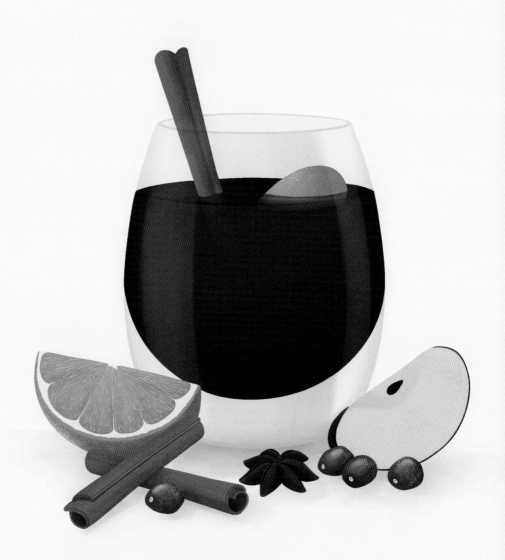

Moringa Mulled Wine

Prized for its nutritional density, moringa is an adaptogenic ingredient that has been used as a traditional herbal medicine for centuries by many Southeast Asian countries. High in vitamin C (it contains seven times the amount found in oranges) and rich in calcium, iron, and magnesium, among other essential minerals, you can see why this native Indian plant is so important to these cultures.

As an adaptogen, moringa is an important ally in fighting cognitive decline; the antioxidants found in the leaves of the plant may even be helpful in treating diseases such as dementia and Alzheimer's disease. To up the adaptogenic power here, included in the recipe is a wee dram of gotu kola to assist with stress, anxiety, and detoxification.

To make this festive, wintery, Wine-NO drink, I've paired the moringa and gotu kola with another vitamin C–rich ingredient: cranberry, a great immune booster. Culinarily speaking, it's most often partnered with sweet apple to mitigate the tartness of the berry and make it more palatable. To finish off this holiday offering, a healthy dose of chai spices does the trick to fill both your kitchen and your soul with a wonderful cozy spirit!

FOR THE MORINGA MULLED WINE

1 milliliter (20 drops) moringa extract

2 milliliters (40 drops) gotu kola extract

1½ ounces (45 ml) unsweetened real cranberry juice

1½ ounces (45 ml) red verjus

3 ounces (90 ml) unsweetened apple juice

1 rooibos chai tea bag

½ ounce (15 ml) runny honey (optional)

FOR SERVING

1 cinnamon stick, for garnish (optional)

YIELD: 1 WINE-NO DRINK

TO MAKE THE MORINGA MULLED WINE: Add all the ingredients, including the tea bag, to a small heavy-bottomed pan and place it on the stove over low heat. Allow the mixture to warm through but do not simmer or boil. Let the tea bag steep in the liquid for at least 5 to 10 minutes.

TO SERVE: Remove the tea bag and pour the infused "wine" into a heatproof mug. Garnish with a cinnamon stick if you're feeling fancy.

Golden Turmeric Cream

When I was a kid, Irish cream was a special welcome gift for any visitor we had during the holidays. My Gran would break out her finest crystal liqueur glasses and fill them to the brim with that lush, creamy, legs-for-days nectar, served always with spiced ginger cookies.

By the time I reached drinking age, I'd mostly lost interest in this overly sweet after-dinner drink, but I was curious if it was possible to make it less sugary and more complex. Cut to twenty-five years later, and I was tasked with creating a nonalcoholic version for a Christmas party, which by itself was pretty tasty. Add in some adaptogenic magic, and this booze-free Irish cream becomes really special.

The holidays are not always a time of joy—hello, traveling stress and seasonal depression. I chose turmeric for its mood-stabilizing properties that help counteract depression, as well as the boost it offers to your immune system. I've also included shiitake, which adds its ability to increase virility, youthfulness, and energy, making this a delightful dessert drink or toast maker!

FOR THE GOLDEN TURMERIC CREAM

1 tablespoon (20 g) chopped fresh peeled turmeric root or 2 tablespoons (30 g) ground turmeric

Scant 1 ounce (30 ml) shiitake extract

1 cup (8 oz or 235 ml) plant-based milk of your choice

3 cups (24 oz or 710 ml) plant-based creamer of your choice

1 cup (8 oz or 235 ml) cold brew or chilled espresso

4 ounces (120 ml) Grade-A Vermont maple syrup

2 milliliters (40 drops) real vanilla extract

1 healthy pinch of sea salt

FOR SERVING

Freshly grated nutmeg

YIELD: ABOUT 15 SERVINGS

TO MAKE THE GOLDEN TURMERIC CREAM: Add all the ingredients to your blender and blend on high for 30 seconds. Strain though a fine-mesh strainer. Allow the bubbles to settle before serving.

TO SERVE: Pour into chilled glasses and sprinkle with nutmeg.

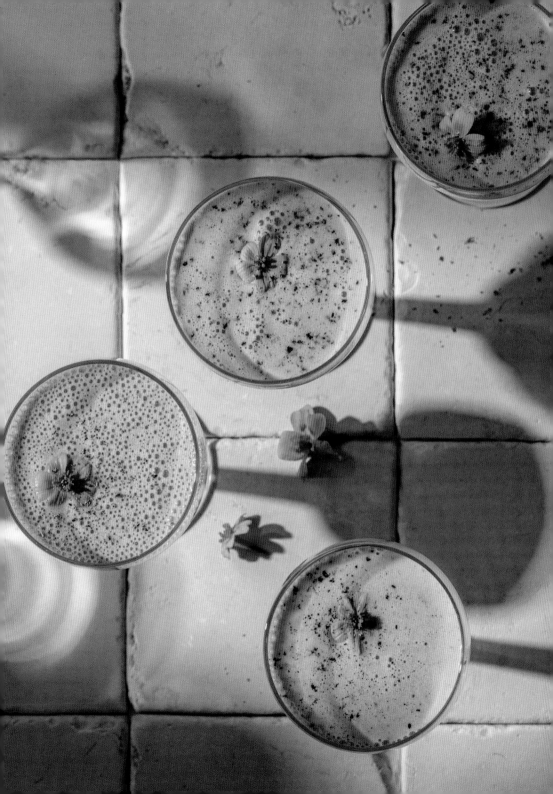

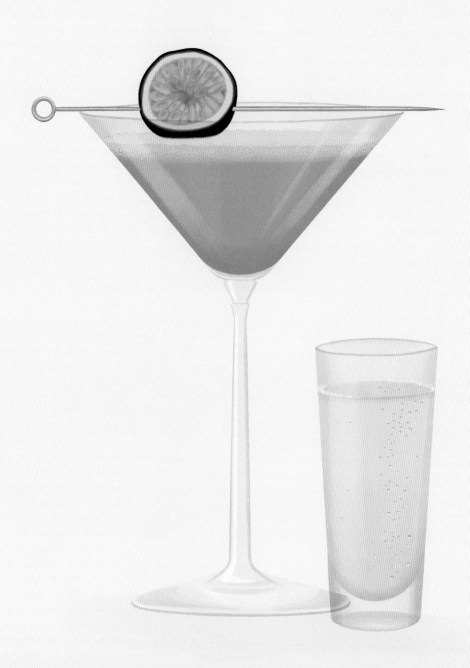

Maca-Tini

This recipe is inspired by a classic cocktail called the Porn Star Martini, created by bartending legend Douglas Ankrah. Invented in 2002, he so named it because he felt it was a cocktail that porn stars would drink. The name may be a bit tasteless, but the cocktail is anything but, combining passion fruit puree, a measure of booze, and bubbly wine. The booze-free version is just as incredible (you had me at passion fruit).

The adaptogens I chose for my re-christened maca-tini, are maca, obviously, for its mood-enhancing and immune-boosting properties, and ashwagandha, to help calm the mind and aid with sleep. Drink it straight up without the bubbly or add your choice of either sparkling nonalcoholic wine, cider, soda water, ginger beer, or even kombucha, depending on the occasion. Personally, I love to serve Maca-tinis for celebratory events—after all, why should nondrinkers miss out on all the festive fun?

FOR THE MACA-TINI

1 milliliter (20 drops)
maca extract

0.7 milliliter (14 drops)
ashwagandha extract

1 ounce (30 ml)
passion fruit puree

½ ounce (15 ml) fresh-squeezed
lime juice

2 ounces (60 ml) chilled mango
iced tea or caffeine-free tea of
your choice

1 drop real vanilla extract

FOR SERVING

1 ounce (30 ml) nonalcoholic
bubbly wine or sparkling cider
(optional)

YIELD: 1 NO-CKTAIL

TO MAKE THE MACA-TINI: Add all the ingredients with 5 ice cubes to your cocktail shaker or mason jar with a lid. Shake hard for 10 seconds. Strain into a chilled coupe or martini glass.

TO SERVE: To enjoy with the bubbly wine or cider on the side, serve it in a shot glass or pour it directly into the cocktail for a fizzy drink.

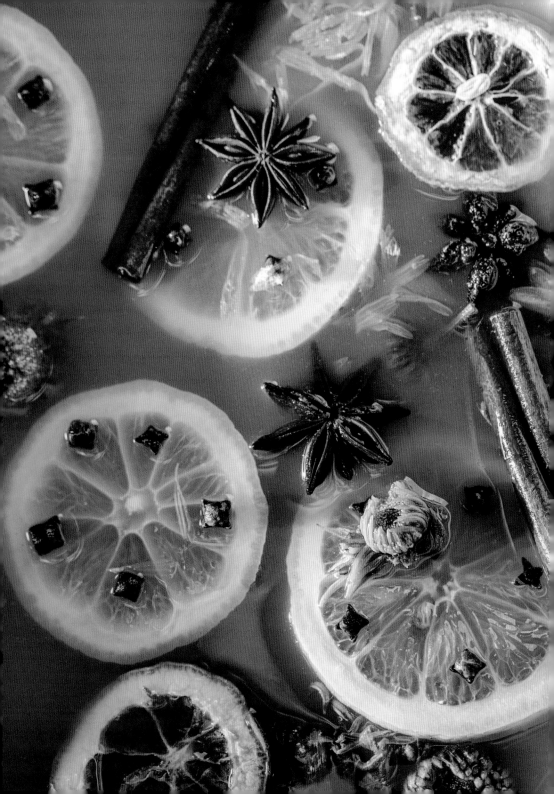

Schisandra–Brown Butter Wassail

The tradition of wassail goes back to ancient England. In this Yuletide drinking ritual, large steaming pots of a warming brew were made by communities and taken door to door as a salutation to ensure a good harvest the following year. The recipe featured hot mulled cider or wine, spices, herbs, and other fruits.

In this adaptogenic version, I use schisandra berry extract for its ability to quell anxiety, as well as boost immunity and endurance, and maca, known for its mood-enhancing properties. For a touch of holiday decadence, brown butter is whipped into the hot fruity mix to make it full to the brim with yummy feel-good vibes. Warm, tart, and just a little spicy, this wassail is the perfect way to come together and celebrate the holiday season.

**FOR THE LIQUID
BROWN BUTTER**

½ pound (227 g)
unsalted butter, cubed

**FOR THE SCHISANDRA–
BROWN BUTTER WASSAIL**

3¾ cups (30 oz or 900 ml)
fresh-pressed apple cider

5 ounces (150 ml) Grade-A
Vermont maple syrup

5 ounces (150 ml) fresh-
squeezed lemon juice

10 whole cinnamon sticks

5 star anise pods

20 whole cloves

10 dried calendula flowers or
dried chamomile flowers

5 slices peeled fresh ginger root

10 thin slices lemon

¼ cup (24 g) dried orange peel

2 to 3 bay leaves

continued on next page

YIELD: 10 SERVINGS

TO MAKE THE LIQUID BROWN BUTTER: Add the butter to a heavy-bottomed saucepan over low heat. Let the butter melt, stirring constantly. The butter will start to bubble; this is the water evaporating, which is what you want!

Once the water has evaporated, the milk solids will start to caramelize and turn brown very quickly. Keep a close watch on this and continue stirring; the milk solids can go from amber to brown to black in seconds, and once they're black, the butter is burnt and unusable.

When the butter is a golden-brown color, remove it from the heat. Allow it to cool slightly before whipping it into the wassail.

TO MAKE THE SCHISANDRA–BROWN BUTTER WASSAIL: Add all the ingredients to a large, lidded, cast-iron pan over low heat. Let the wassail come up to a low simmer, then reduce the heat and cover with the lid, allowing all the lovely flavors to infuse for at least 1 hour.

continued on next page

2 ounces (60 ml)
Liquid Brown Butter

4 teaspoons (400 drops or
20 ml) schisandra berry extract

2 teaspoons (200 drops or
10 ml) maca extract

Clove-studded lemon wheels

TO SERVE: Remove the wassail from the heat. Add the liquid brown butter, schisandra berry extract, and maca extract. Use a milk frother (see Note) to whip everything together, making sure the butter is well incorporated. Serve in heatproof punch glasses, and garnish each with a clove-studded lemon wheel.

NOTE
It's important that you use a milk frother, not an immersion blender, in this recipe, as an immersion blender will chop up the lemon, ginger, and flowers.

PRO TIP
I make extra brown butter and store it in the fridge for all manner of dishes, from brown butter ice cream and brown butter maple syrup to sauces for pasta and veggies. Stored in the fridge, it will last a couple of months; you'll just need to melt it before using.

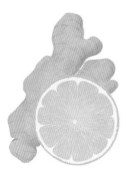

Goji Berry Glogg

Glogg is a heated Scandinavian punch served in the colder months, made from red wine and spices. In this recipe, we're taking out the wine and swapping in pomegranate and blood orange juices, then adding a tropical note by adding pineapple juice, cloves, orange blossom, and vanilla (ingredients often used in tiki-style cocktails).

As for adaptogens, my choices here are goji berry and velvet bean. Goji berry is a great immune support and anti-inflammatory that is packed with vitamins A, C, and B, as well as magnesium and zinc. The velvet bean contains high concentrations of L-dopa, the precursor of dopamine, and it is a fantastic defense against anxiety and depression.

Once you've made the syrup component, this recipe comes together fairly quickly, but it gets better the longer you allow the spices to infuse the liquid. Make a batch and keep it in your fridge all holiday season for a heartwarming draught of wintery cheer!

FOR THE FALERNUM SYRUP

2 cups (454 g) demerara sugar (see Pro Tip)

2 cups (16 oz or 475 ml) hot water

½ ounce (15 ml) good-quality almond extract

½ ounce (15 ml) real vanilla extract

1 ounce (30 ml) orange blossom water

20 whole cloves

4 dried black limes (Buy them online; their fragrance is intoxicating.)

continued on next page

continued on next page

YIELD: 10 SERVINGS

TO MAKE THE FALERNUM SYRUP: Add all the ingredients to a heavy-bottomed pan and place it over low heat. Let the mixture heat through, while stirring constantly, about 10 minutes, until the sugar is fully dissolved. Do not let the syrup reach a simmer or boil or the sugar will burn.

When the sugar is dissolved, remove the syrup from the heat, transfer it to an airtight container, and store in the fridge. Allow the syrup to steep for up to 5 days in the fridge to get the fullest extraction of flavors from the dried black limes and cloves. After that, store it in the fridge for up to 2 months.

TO MAKE THE GOJI BERRY GLOGG: Add all the ingredients to a large, lidded, heavy-bottomed pan or Dutch oven. Place the pan over medium-low heat and heat the glogg until just before the liquid comes to a simmer, about 10 minutes. Place a lid on the pan and reduce the heat to the lowest it will go. Allow the glogg to steep for up to 1 hour.

continued on next page

FOR THE GOJI BERRY GLOGG

2½ cups (20 oz or 570 ml) unsweetened pomegranate juice

5 ounces (150 ml) fresh-squeezed blood orange juice

1¼ cups (10 oz or 285 ml) unsweetened pineapple juice

1¼ cups (10 oz or 285 ml) Falernum Syrup

10 whole cinnamon sticks

10 whole cloves

FOR SERVING

2 teaspoons (200 drops or 10 ml) velvet bean extract (see Note)

1¼ cups (10 oz or 285 ml) Goji Berry Juice (page 55)

Dried orange slices

1 tablespoon (14 g) whole pink peppercorns

TO SERVE: Add the adaptogens and give it a good stir. Serve in heatproof toddy mugs and garnish with a dried orange slice and pink peppercorns.

PRO TIP
Falernum syrup is a staple of tiki cocktails, usually fortified with Jamaican rum. I use demerara sugar to imitate the flavor profile. You can use falernum syrup in all manner of beverages. Swap it in for simple syrup to gussy up a simple soda water, limeade, or alcohol-free mojito.

NOTE
Velvet bean is often labeled as *Mucuna pruriens*.

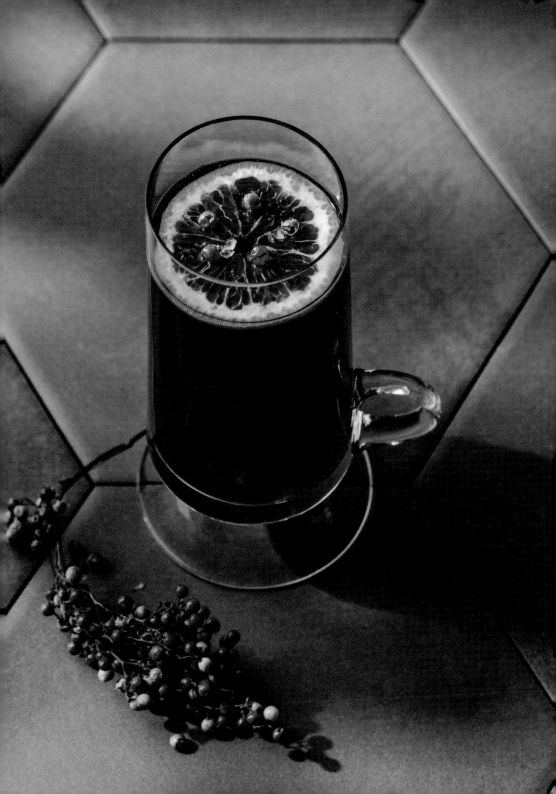

Recipe List by Adaptogen

Lion's Mane

"Mind Embracer" Lion's Mane Mule	38
Lion's Mane Vietnamese Coffee	63
"In Like a Lion" Serotonin Shot	110
"Do the Mochamotion" Mushroom Latte	128

Maca

Maca Garden Greens Shot	42
The Maca Fauxito	47
"Pinkies Out" Amla Sour	64
Turmeric Maca Paleta	82
Mango Maca Lassi	92
No-Bull Energy Shot	108
Reishi & Maca "Sleepy Time" Cosmo	114
You Maca Me Crazy! Sour	137
Maca-Tini	149
Schisandra–Brown Butter Wassail	151

Moringa

Ashwagandha White Grape Bianco Aperitivo	44
Sandíalada	86
PPP Moringa Spritz	98
Moringa Unicorn Latte	112
You Maca Me Crazy! Sour	137
Moringa Mulled Wine	145

Nettle

Maca Garden Greens Shot	42

Pine Pollen

Matcha, Matcha, Matcha!	26
Silver Needle Schisandra Shot	41
Hocus Focus Shot	73
Apple Pine Pollen Shake	91
Big Boost Banana Smoothie	124

Reishi

Relaxing Reishi Tisane	51
Eastern Crush	84
Mushroom Morning Glory Latte	96
Reishi & Maca "Sleepy Time" Cosmo	114
"Do the Mochamotion" Mushroom Latte	128
Reishi Ginger Nightcap	143

Rhodiola

Jolly Green Rhodiola Smoothie	28
Holy Rhodiola Smoothie Bowl (or Acai Bowl)	58
Goji Berry Go-Go Shot	78
Fuzzy Navel Punch with Rhodiola	85

Vie en Rose "Margarita" with Holy Basil	100
No-Bull Energy Shot	108
The MVP Shot	142

Schisandra Berry

Silver Needle Schisandra Shot	41
Schisandra Berry Peachy Palmer	61
Schisandra Shandy	67
Apple Pine Pollen Shake	91
Superberry Punch	119
Sangresandra "Margarita"	133
Schisandra–Brown Butter Wassail	151

Sea Buckthorn

Schisandra Berry Peachy Palmer	61
Frosé All Day	79
Sea Buck Immunity Shot	139

Shatavari

Shatavari "Salty Dog"	35
Shatavari Champagne Spritz	70
Sandíalada	86
Turmeric Shatavari Zinger	105
Morning, Sunshine! Gotu Kola Toddy	127

Shiitake

Shiitake Almond Mocha Rocha	29
Mushroom Morning Glory Latte	96
Rosy Glow Horchata with Shiitake & Velvet Bean	120
"Do the Mochamotion" Mushroom Latte	128
Bacopa Cup-a-Soup	140
Golden Turmeric Cream	146

Turmeric

"Going for Gold!" Turmeric Shot	43
Schisandra Shandy	67
Turmeric Maca Paleta	82
Dirty Chaga Chai	95
Turmeric Shatavari Zinger	105
Rising Sun Shake	130
Turmeric Buck	134
Golden Turmeric Cream	146

Velvet Bean

Velvet Bean Shake	60
Rosy Glow Horchata with Shiitake & Velvet Bean	120
Ashitaba Energy Booster	138
Goji Berry Glogg	153

Acknowledgments

A thousand thanks to Nicola Parisi for being such a great partner in creative crimes and for turning this around so quickly, and to Julia Bainbridge for connecting the dots. I'd also like to thank my editor Hilary for making this process so easy!

About the Author

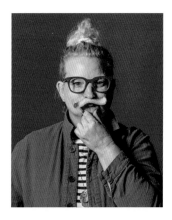

Award-winning bartender, bar director, and mixologist Gaby Mlynarczyk has been reinventing cocktails and how we drink for the last twenty years, working alongside some of the best chefs in America and learning their tricks on flavor balance. Her beverage and bar programs have won numerous awards from *Time Out, Eater, L.A. Times*, and James Beard. She is the author of *Clean + Dirty Drinking* (Chronicle Books, 2018) and has written for *LA Weekly, New York Post, Liquor*, and *Gather* journal as well as her blog, *The Loving Cup*. She has been an avid proponent of nonalcoholic cocktails since 2013. When not mixing beverages, Gaby serves as a brand ambassador for Future Gin, a woman and queer-owned distillery in Los Angeles, Caifornia, teaches ceramics, and works as a food stylist.

Index